MIGRAINE MASTERCLASS:
Your Comprehensive Guide to Understanding, Managing, and Conquering Headaches.

By
Cynthia E. Cortez.

<u>Copyright</u>

All rights reserved. No part of this publication may be reproduced, distributed, or transmitted in any form or by any means, including photocopying, recording, or other electronic or mechanical methods, without the prior written permission of the publisher, except in the case of brief quotations embodied in critical reviews and certain other noncommercial uses permitted by copyright law.

Copyright © Cynthia E. Cortez, 2023.

Table Of Content

CHAPTER 1

<u>AN INTRODUCTION TO MIGRAINES</u>

HISTORIA DE LAS MIGRANAS

In the dimly lighted corridors of history, there resides a narrative of anguish and mystery, one that has afflicted mankind for centuries—the intriguing saga of migraines. Imagine yourself transported back in time, to an age when the pulsing ache in your brain had no name, and the cures were as perplexing as the sickness itself.

Our trip starts in ancient times, when the earliest documented reports of migraines trace back to the Mesopotamians, approximately 4,000 years ago. These ancient people defined their pounding headaches as "the demon who takes over," a suitable metaphor for a sickness that might seem like a malicious force at work. In ancient times, migraines were commonly ascribed to supernatural origins, with demonic possession, curses, or even offended gods being blamed for the misery.

As the ages passed, our knowledge of migraines steadily changed. The Greeks, for example, thought that headaches were a consequence of an imbalance in the body's four humors, leading to odd therapies such as bloodletting and the consumption of foul-tasting concoctions.

The Roman physician Galen, famed for his breakthrough work on medicine, contributed by stating that migraines came from a malfunction in the cranial veins, an idea that fits with contemporary vascular theories.

The idea of "aura" in migraines, a word used by the Greek physician Hippocrates, provided another degree of mysticism. Auras are sensory disturbances that precede or follow a migraine episode, and they might show as visual disturbances, such as flashing lights or zigzag lines. In ancient times, these auras were commonly considered as omens or otherworldly visions, further strengthening the mystical relationship between migraines and the unknown.

Fast forward to the medieval age, and we find ourselves among a multitude of quirky migraine cures. Some thought that putting a piece of freshly cut raw onion to the temples would reduce the agony, while others advocated for the usage of medicines and amulets to fight against bad spirits. In an age when science and superstition entwined, it's no wonder that migraine sufferers clutched at any possible cure, no matter how unusual.

The Renaissance brought with it the blooming of medical knowledge, and doctors started to investigate more logical methods for migraines. Still, therapies remained far from current norms.

Physicians like Ambroise Paré, a French surgeon from the 16th century, experimented with therapies including trepanation, a process requiring drilling holes into the skull to remove pressure. Though this procedure sounds barbarous now, it was a sincere endeavor to understand and relieve migraine symptoms.

It wasn't until the 19th and early 20th century that migraine therapy began to take on a more scientific and humane tone. Pioneers in neurology, such as Sir William Gowers and Sigmund Freud, started to probe into the psychological and neurological elements of migraines, opening the door for more successful treatment options.

In the contemporary period, our knowledge of migraines has gone a long way. Thanks to breakthroughs in neuroscience, we now know that migraines are a complicated neurological illness, with many causes and hereditary components. Treatments have developed to include drugs that help prevent or treat migraine episodes, coupled with lifestyle adjustments and behavioral therapy.

The history of migraines is a monument to humanity's constant desire for knowledge and comfort. From the mystical beliefs of ancient civilizations to the odd remedies of the medieval period, the tale of migraines is one of perseverance in the face of agonizing agony.

As we continue to uncover the intricacies of this perplexing ailment, let us remember the numerous people throughout history who had migraines and the often bizarre remedies that came with them, each step bringing us closer to the understanding and relief we enjoy today.

WHAT IS AN AURA?

An aura is a combination of sensory, motor, and verbal symptoms that generally behave as warning signs that a migraine headache is about to begin. Commonly misunderstood as a seizure or stroke, it normally comes before the headache pain, but may also arise during or even after. An aura might endure from 10 to 60 minutes. About 15% to 20% of persons who get migraines have auras.

Aura symptoms are reversible, meaning that they may be stopped/healed. An aura creates symptoms that may include:

- Seeing brilliant flashing dots, sparkles, or lights.
- Blind areas in your eyesight.
- Numb or tingling skin.
- Speech changes.
- Ringing in your ears (tinnitus).
- Temporary eyesight loss.
- Seeing wavy or jagged lines.
- Changes in scent or flavor.
- A "funny" sensation.

EXPLORING THE SCIENCE OF MIGRAINES

The brain, the most fascinating organ in our body, is the cornerstone of a migraine. It serves as a control center, sending and receiving information to make sure that all areas of our body are operating correctly. When a migraine develops, something interferes with this symphony and the brain starts to malfunction.

The trigeminal nerve, which is responsible for sensation in the face, is a crucial component in the migraine drama.
It sends messages to the blood vessels surrounding the brain to constrict and then expand, which leads to an increase in pain when it senses anything wrong, such as specific meals, stress, or hormonal changes.

The throbbing anguish that migraineurs are all too acquainted with is generated by these fluctuations in blood flow, which function as crescendos in the migraine symphony.

Neurotransmitters, the messengers that convey impulses between nerve cells, are also crucial components of the brain. Serotonin, a neurotransmitter that helps govern mood and pain perception, is one of the primary causes.
During a migraine episode, serotonin levels in patients change considerably, bringing off those terrible crescendos in the migraine symphony.

The aura is another intriguing character in this narrative. Although not all migraineurs experience it, for those who do, it works as a prologue to the main event.

Auras may appear as visual disturbances like zigzag or flashing lights, or they might feel tingling in the limbs. Scientists think that these auras are created by a transient increase in aberrant electrical activity in the brain, which is like a lightning storm in the depths of your mind.

Genetics may potentially be an influence on migraines. Since migraines commonly run in families, this neurological disorder may have a genetic origin. Researchers have found particular genes associated with migraines, and these genes may impact a person's susceptibility to outside stimuli. It's as if some folks possessed a more sensitive symphony, where even a slight interruption may produce pandemonium.

Finally, inflammation may be the culmination of our migraine saga. Studies have revealed that when a migraine episode happens, the brain is inflamed and produces chemicals that make the agony considerably worse. This inflammation may be yet another impact of the brain's hypersensitivity, which makes it look as though it is responding to perceived hazards.

Migraines are a complicated dance involving the trigeminal nerve, serotonin, auras, genetics, and inflammation that frequently leaves migraine patients yearning for a solution. We have made enormous progress in our knowledge of this enigmatic condition, but there is still much to learn about the ever-evolving history of migraines.

WHAT KIND OF HEADACHES ARE THERE, AND WHAT KIND OF HEADACHES IS A MIGRAINE?

At some moment in their lives, practically everyone may suffer headaches, which are a common ailment. They drastically impact our regular lives and may cause anything from slight pain to major misery. Effective management and treatment of headaches relies on having a good awareness of the many kinds and their distinct characteristics. This section will discuss several varieties of headaches, with a focus on migraines, and potential remedies.

TYPES OF HEADACHES

TENSION HEADACHES:
CHARACTERISTICS: Tension headaches are the most prevalent form of headache. They typically feel like a continual ring of pressure around the head.

CAUSES: Stress, muscular strain, poor posture, and exhaustion are major causes.

TREATMENT: Over-the-counter pain medications, relaxation methods, and treating the underlying causes including stress management and better posture will help eliminate tension headaches.

CLUSTER HEADACHES:
CHARACTERISTICS: Cluster headaches are painfully painful and generally recur in clusters over weeks or months.

CAUSES: The specific cause is uncertain, however, they may be connected to anomalies in the hypothalamus.

TREATMENT: Oxygen therapy, triptans, and preventative medicines may be beneficial in controlling cluster headaches.

SINUS HEADACHES:
CHARACTERISTICS: Sinus headaches are commonly coupled with sinus congestion and face discomfort, often caused by sinusitis.

CAUSES: Inflammation and inflammation of the sinuses.

TREATMENT: Treating the underlying sinus disease with antibiotics or decongestants may reduce sinus headaches.

REBOUND HEADACHES:
CHARACTERISTICS: Rebound headaches arise when overusing pain drugs leads to a pattern of repeated headaches.

CAUSES: Frequent use of pain medications, particularly those containing caffeine or opioids.

TREATMENT: Gradual removal from the overused medicine, along with lifestyle modifications and alternate pain management measures, is crucial.

MIGRAINE HEADACHES

Migraines are a specific form of headache marked by strong, throbbing pain, frequently on one side of the head.
They are frequently accompanied by additional symptoms such as nausea, vomiting, sensitivity to light and sound, and aura (visual abnormalities). Migraines may be classified into two primary types:

Migraine Without Aura: This is the most frequent kind when migraine episodes occur without any distinct warning symptoms. The agony might linger for hours to days.

Migraine With Aura: Some persons feel "auras" before or during a migraine. Auras are frequently visual disruptions like flashing lights or zigzag lines. These indications might help patients prepare for the oncoming migraine.

Causes Of Migraines:
The specific origin of migraines is still not entirely known, although various variables might trigger them, including genetics, hormone swings, environmental conditions, and particular foods.

Treatment For Migraines:
Migraine therapy often comprises a mix of lifestyle modifications, preventative measures, and acute treatments:

Lifestyle Changes: Identifying and avoiding migraine triggers, such as particular meals, stress, and lack of sleep, might help lessen the frequency and intensity of attacks.

Preventive drugs: In situations of frequent or severe migraines, physicians may prescribe drugs to avoid attacks. These may include beta-blockers, anticonvulsants, and botulinum toxin injections.

Acute Treatments: When a migraine episode develops, acute treatments such as triptans or nonsteroidal anti-inflammatory drugs (NSAIDs) might help reduce pain and other symptoms.

Lifestyle Remedies: Resting in a quiet, dark room, putting cold packs on the forehead, and keeping hydrated may also give comfort during a migraine.

Headaches exist in numerous forms, each with its distinct features and causes. Among them, migraines stand out owing to their extreme pain and related symptoms. Understanding the kind of headache you are having is vital for optimal treatment and management. If you routinely get severe headaches, visit a healthcare expert for a correct diagnosis and individualized treatment plan, since treating headaches may considerably improve your quality of life.

WHAT ARE THE TYPES OF MIGRAINES?

There are various varieties of migraines, and the same type may go by multiple names:

Migraine with aura (complex migraine): Around 15% to 20% of persons with migraine symptoms get an aura.

MIGRAINE WITHOUT AURA (common migraine): This form of migraine headache hits without the warning that aura may offer you. The symptoms are the same, but that period doesn't happen.

MIGRAINE WITHOUT HEAD PAIN: "Silent migraine" or "acephalgic migraine," as this form is often known, contains the aura symptom but without the headache that normally follows.

HEMIPLEGIC MIGRAINE: You'll experience momentary paralysis (hemiplegia) or neurological or sensory alterations on one side of your body.
The development of the headache may be coupled with momentary numbness, acute weakness on one side of your body, a tingling feeling, a loss of sensation, and dizziness or visual problems. Sometimes it involves head discomfort and sometimes it doesn't.

RETINAL MIGRAINE (ocular migraine): You may experience brief, partial, or total loss of vision in one of your eyes, combined with a dull aching behind the eye that may extend to the rest of your head. That visual loss may last a minute, or as long as months. You should always report a retinal migraine to a healthcare physician since it might be an indication of a more severe condition.

CHRONIC MIGRAINE: A chronic migraine is a migraine that occurs at least 15 days a month. The symptoms may fluctuate regularly, and so may the level of the discomfort.
Those who have chronic migraines could be utilizing headache pain drugs more than 10 to 15 days a month and that, regrettably, might contribute to headaches that come even more often.

MIGRAINE WITH BRAINSTEM AURA:
With this migraine, you'll experience vertigo, slurred speech, double vision, or loss of balance, which comes before the headache. The headache discomfort may impact the back of your head. These symptoms frequently arise quickly and might be coupled with the inability to talk correctly, ringing in the ears, and vomiting.

STATUS MIGRAINOSUS: This is an uncommon and severe kind of migraine that may persist for longer than 72 hours. The headache pain and nausea might be really intense. Certain drugs, or medication withdrawal, might cause you to experience this form of migraine.

WHAT ARE THE FOUR STAGES OR PHASES OF A MIGRAINE? WHAT'S THE TIMELINE?

The four phases in chronological sequence are the prodrome (pre-monitory), aura, headache, and postdrome. About 30% of individuals feel symptoms before their headache begins.

The stages are:

PRODROME: The initial stage lasts a few hours, although it might last days. You may or may not experience it since it may not happen every time. Some recognize it as the "preheadache" or "premonitory" period.

AURA: The aura phase might last as long as 60 minutes or as little as five. Most individuals don't feel an aura, and others have both the aura and the headache at the same time.

HEADACHE: About four hours to 72 hours is how long the headache lasts. The phrase "ache" doesn't do the agony credit since occasionally it's minor, but frequently, it's characterized as drilling, throbbing, or you may experience the feeling of an icepick in your brain. Typically it begins on one side of your head and then travels to the other side.

POSTDROME: The postdrome stage continues on for a day or two. It's sometimes dubbed a migraine "hangover" and 80% of individuals who get migraines experience it.
It might take around eight to 72 hours to get through the four phases.

HOW COMMON ARE MIGRAINE HEADACHES?

Experts estimate that over half of the adult population has headaches and 12% of Americans have migraine headaches. Women are nearly three times as likely than males to get migraines.

WHO GETS MIGRAINES? WHAT ARE THE RISK FACTORS?

It's impossible to predict who may have a migraine and who may not, but there are risk factors that may make you more sensitive. These risk factors include:

GENETICS: Up to 80% of persons who experience migraine headaches have a first-degree relative with the condition.

GENDER: Migraine headaches occurs in women more than males, particularly women between the ages of 15 and 55. It's presumably more frequent in women because of the effect of hormones.

STRESS LEVEL: You may suffer migraines more frequently if you're high-stress. Stress might provoke a migraine.
Smoking.

HOW OFTEN DO MIGRAINES HAPPEN?

The frequency of a migraine might be once a year, once a week, or any length of time in between. Having two to four migraine headaches each month is the most frequent.

ARE MIGRAINES HEREDITARY?

Migraines tend to run in families. As many as four out of five persons with migraines have a familial history. If one parent has a history of migraines, their kid has a 50% risk of experiencing them. If both parents have a history of migraines, the risk climbs to 75%. Again, up to 80% of persons with migraines have a first-degree family with the condition.

CAN CHILDREN GET MIGRAINES?

Yes, although pediatric migraines are frequently shorter and there are more stomach symptoms.

WHO SHOULD I SEE ABOUT MY MIGRAINE PAIN?

Discuss your symptoms with your primary care provider first. They may identify migraine headaches and start therapy. You may need a referral to a headache specialist.

DO MIGRAINES CAUSE PERMANENT BRAIN DAMAGE? IF I HAVE MIGRAINES, DOES THAT MEAN I'LL GET ANOTHER DISEASE?

No. Migraines don't cause brain damage. There is a modest risk of stroke in persons who experience migraines with aura — 1 or 2 people out of 100,000.

SYMPTOMS AND CAUSES

What Are The Symptoms Of Migraines?

The main symptom of migraine is a headache. Pain is frequently characterized as hammering or throbbing. It might begin as a dull aching that escalates into pulsating pain that is mild, moderate, or severe. If left untreated, your headache pain will develop moderate to severe. Pain might vary from one side of your head to the other, or it can impact the front of your head, the rear of your head, or seem like it's hurting your entire head. Some patients experience discomfort around their eye or temple, and occasionally in their face, sinuses, jaw, or neck.

Other Signs Of Migraine Headaches Include:
- Sensitivity to light, noise, and scents.
- Nausea and vomiting, upset stomach, and abdominal discomfort.
- Loss of appetite.
- Feeling excessively heated (sweating) or freezing (chills).
- Pale skin hue (pallor).
- Feeling exhausted.
- Dizziness and hazy eyesight.

- Tender scalp.
- Diarrhea (rare).
- Fever (rare).
- Most migraines last approximately four hours, while severe ones might last considerably longer.

Each Phase Of The Migraine Episode Might Come With Distinct Symptoms:

Prodrome Symptoms:
- Problems focusing.
- Irritability and/or sadness.
- Difficulty speaking and reading.
- Difficulty sleeping. Yawning.
- Nausea.
- Fatigue.
- Sensitivity to light and sound.
- Food desires.
- Increased urination.
- Muscle tightness.

Aura Symptoms:

- Numbness and tingling.
- Visual disturbances. You could be viewing the world as though through a kaleidoscope, have hazy areas, or see sparkles or lines.
- Temporary loss of sight.
- Weakness on one side of the body.
- Speech changes.

Headache Symptoms:
- Neck ache, stiffness.
- Depression, giddiness, and/or anxiousness.
- Sensitivity to light, scent, and sound.
- Nasal congestion.
- Insomnia.
- Nausea and vomiting.

Postdrome Symptoms:
- Inability to focus.
- Depressed mood.
- Fatigue.
- Lack of understanding.
- Euphoric mood.

WHAT CAUSES A MIGRAINE?

The etiology of migraine headaches is multifaceted and not entirely understood. When you develop a headache it's because certain neurons in your blood vessels deliver pain messages to your brain. This releases inflammatory molecules into the nerves and blood vessels of your brain. It's unknown why your nerves do that.

WHAT TRIGGERS A MIGRAINE?

Migraine episodes may be induced by a number of circumstances. Common triggers include:

EMOTIONAL TENSION: Emotional tension is one of the most prevalent causes of migraine headaches. During stressful circumstances, specific chemicals in the brain are produced to battle the situation (known as the "flight or fight" reaction). The release of these substances might bring on a migraine. Other emotions like fear, concern, and enthusiasm may raise muscular tension and widen blood vessels. That may make your migraine more acute.

MISSING A LUNCH: Delaying a meal could potentially aggravate your migraine headache.

SENSITIVITY TO PARTICULAR CHEMICALS AND PRESERVATIVES IN MEALS: Certain foods and drinks such as aged cheese, beverages containing alcohol, chocolate and food additives such as nitrates (found in pepperoni, hot dogs, and luncheon meats) and fermented or pickled foods may be responsible for inducing up to 30% of migraines.

CAFFEINE: Having too much caffeine or withdrawal from caffeine might produce headaches when the caffeine level quickly declines. Your blood vessels appear to get reactive to coffee and when you don't receive it, a headache may result. Caffeine is occasionally prescribed by healthcare practitioners to aid in treating acute migraine episodes but should not be taken regularly.

DAILY USAGE OF PAIN-RELIEVING MEDICINES: If you take medication designed to treat headache pain too frequently, it might induce a rebound headache.

HORMONAL CHANGES IN WOMEN: Migraines in women are more prevalent around the time of their monthly cycles. The sudden reduction in estrogen that accompanies menses might also produce migraines. Hormonal alterations may also be brought on by birth control medications and hormone replacement treatment.

Migraines are often worse between puberty and menopause as these estrogen changes normally don't occur in young girls and post-menopausal women. If your hormones have a big impact on your migraines, you may experience fewer headaches after menopause. Hormonal changes do not seem to produce migraines in males.

Light. Flashing lights, fluorescent lights, light from the TV or computer and sunshine might provoke you.

Other probable causes include:

- Changing weather conditions such as storm fronts, barometric pressure fluctuations, severe winds, or changes in altitude.
- Being extremely fatigued. Overexertion.
- Dieting, or not drinking enough water.
- Changes in your typical sleep routine.
- Loud sounds.
- Exposure to smoking, perfumes, or other scents.
- Certain drugs cause blood vessels to enlarge.

DIAGNOSIS AND TESTS

What's a migraine journal?

Keeping a migraine journal is not only useful to you but also assists your healthcare practitioner with the diagnosing process. Your diary should be thorough and updated as much as possible before, during, and after a migraine episode. Consider keeping note of the following:

- The date and time of when the migraine began – especially when the prodrome started if you're able to determine it's occurring. Track time passing. When did the aura phase begin? The headache? The postdrome? Do your best to tell what stage you're in and how long it lasts. If there's a trend, that may assist you in forecasting what will happen in the future.
- What are your symptoms? Be specific.
- Note how many hours of sleep you had the night before it occurred and your stress level. What's causing your stress?

- Note the weather.
- Log your meal and water consumption. Did you consume anything that prompted the migraine? Did you skip a meal?
- Describe the sort of pain and grade it on a one to 10 scale with 10 being the worst pain you've ever experienced.
- Where is the pain located? One side of your head? Your jaw? Your eye?
- List all of the drugs you took. This includes any daily medicines, any vitamins, and any pain medication you use.
- How did you attempt to treat your migraine, and did it work? What drug did you take, at what dose, at what time?
- Consider additional causes. Maybe you played basketball in the sunlight? Maybe you saw a movie that featured flashing lights? If you're a woman, are you on your period?

- There are various smartphone applications you may use to maintain a migraine notebook if you don't want to use pen and paper.

HOW ARE MIGRAINES DIAGNOSED?

To diagnose a migraine, your healthcare professional will gather a detailed medical history, not only your history of headaches but your family's, too. Also, they'll want to construct a history of your migraine-related symptoms, perhaps asking you to:

- Describe your headache symptoms. How severe are they?
- Remember when you receive them. During your menstruation, for example?
- Describe the nature and location of your pain. Is the ache pounding? Pulsing? Throbbing?
- Remember whether anything makes your headache better or worse.

- Tell me how frequently you have migraine headaches.
- Talk about the activities, meals, stresses, or events that may have brought on the migraine.
- Discuss what drugs you use to treat the pain and how frequently you take them.
- Tell how you felt before, during, and after the headache.
- Remember if anybody in your family has migraine headaches.

Your healthcare practitioner may also conduct blood tests and imaging tests (such as a CT scan or an MRI) to make sure there are no other explanations for your headache. An electroencephalogram (EEG) may be ordered to rule out seizures.

WHAT SYMPTOMS MUST YOU HAVE TO BE DIAGNOSED WITH A MIGRAINE?

MIGRAINE WITH AURA (complicated migraine). This is a headache, plus:

- Visual symptoms (seeing spots, sparkles, or lines) or vision loss.
- Sensory complaints (feeling pins and needles, for example).

MIGRAINE WITHOUT AURA (common migraine). A common migraine is a headache and:

- The assaults featured discomfort on one side of your head.
- You've experienced at least five attacks, each lasting between four and 72 hours.

Plus, you've encountered at least one of the following:

- Nausea and/or vomiting.
- Lights irritate you and/or you shun light.

- noises irritate you and/or you avoid noises.

ARE MIGRAINES MISDIAGNOSED?

Sometimes you or your healthcare practitioner may presume that the pain you're experiencing is a sinus headache or a tension-type headache. Show your healthcare professional your migraine diary so that they may understand your specific circumstance.

MANAGEMENT AND TREATMENT

How Are Migraines Treated?

Migraine headaches are persistent. They can't be healed, but they can be controlled and potentially improved. There are two basic treatment techniques that employ medications: abortive and preventative.

Abortive drugs are most helpful when you take them at the earliest symptoms of a migraine. Take them when the discomfort is modest. By potentially interrupting the headache process, abortive drugs can stop or minimize your migraine symptoms, including pain, nausea, light sensitivity, etc. Some abortive drugs work by narrowing your blood vessels, bringing them back to normal, and reducing the pounding discomfort.

Preventive (prophylactic) drugs may be provided when your headaches are severe, occur more than four times a month, and are considerably interfering with your daily activities. Preventive drugs minimize the frequency and intensity of the headaches. Medications are often given on a regular, daily basis to help avoid migraines.

WHAT DRUGS ARE USED TO ALLEVIATE MIGRAINE PAIN?

Over-the-counter drugs are beneficial for some persons with mild to severe migraines. The major constituents in pain-reducing drugs include ibuprofen, aspirin, acetaminophen, naproxen, and caffeine.

Three over-the-counter medications authorized by the Food and Drug Administration for migraine headaches are:

- Excedrin® Migraine.
- Advil® Migraine.
- Motrin® Migraine Pain.

Be careful while using over-the-counter pain relief drugs. Sometimes overusing them might produce analgesic-rebound headaches or a dependence issue. If you're using any over-the-counter pain drugs more than two to three times a week, mention it to your healthcare physician. They may offer prescription drugs that may be more effective.

Prescription Medications For Migraine Headaches Include:
Triptan family of medicines (these are abortives):

- Sumatriptan.
- Zolmitriptan.
- Naratriptan.

Calcium channel blockers:
- Verapamil.

Calcitonin gene-related (CGRP) monoclonal antibodies:
- Erenumab.
- Fremanezumab.
- Galcanezumab.
- Eptinezumab.

Beta-blockers:
- Atenolol.
- Propranolol.
- Nadolol.

Antidepressants:
- Amitriptyline.
- Nortriptyline.
- Doxepin.
- Venlafaxine.

- Duloxetine.

Antiseizure drugs:
- Valproic acid.
- Topiramate.

Other:
- Steroids.
- Phenothiazines.
- Corticosteroids.

Your healthcare practitioner could suggest vitamins, minerals, or herbs, including:

- Riboflavin (vitamin B2).
- Magnesium.
- Feverfew.
- Butterbur.
- Co-enzyme Q10.

Drugs to treat migraine discomfort exist in a range of forms including pills, tablets, injections, suppositories, and nasal sprays. You and your healthcare practitioner will discuss the particular drug, mix of medications, and formulations to best satisfy your individual headache discomfort.

Drugs to treat nausea are also administered if required.

All drugs should be used under the advice of a headache specialist or healthcare practitioner skilled in migraine management. As with any medicine, it's vital to carefully follow the label directions and your healthcare provider's recommendations.

Alternative migraine care options, usually known as home remedies, include:

- Resting in a dark, quiet, cold place.
- Apply a cold compress or washcloth to your forehead or behind your neck. (Some folks enjoy heat.)
- Massaging your scalp.
- Yoga.

- Applying pressure to your temples in a circular manner.
- Keeping oneself in a peaceful condition. Meditating.

WHAT'S BIOFEEDBACK?

Biofeedback is the use of specific equipment attached to your head. The technology detects the physical tension in your body and informs you when you need to regulate your stress, which modifies the physical processes associated with stress. You won't have to utilize the equipment forever since you'll learn how to identify the stress on your own. The gadget works on youngsters as well as adults.

ARE THERE SURGICAL PROCEDURES THAT RELIEVE MIGRAINES?

Surgical therapies are not normally suggested for migraine headaches.

WHAT ARE THE TREATMENT OPTIONS FOR MIGRAINE HEADACHES DURING PREGNANCY?

Avoid drugs for migraines while you're pregnant, or if you believe you may be pregnant. They may badly impact your baby. With your healthcare provider's authorization, you may be allowed to use a light pain medication like acetaminophen.

MANAGING MIGRAINES DURING PREGNANCY

A magnificent journey, pregnancy is a time of enormous anticipation and change. However, this delightful season may also bring on a hailstorm of headaches for people who are prone to migraines. Pregnancy makes migraine treatment a delicate art of balancing the requirements of mother and child.

Migraines are distinct from typical headaches in many ways. In addition to symptoms like nausea, vomiting, and sensitivity to light and sound, they may be incapacitating, throbbing, and debilitating. Imagine combating them while facing the emotional and physical upheaval of pregnancy! Although it may seem challenging, we are here to assist you in navigating the labyrinth of migraine care during this particular era.

UNDERSTANDING THE CONUNDRUM OF MIGRAINE AND PREGNANCY
Priorities aside, it's vital to realize that while pregnancy could give relief for some migraineurs, it might make the sickness worse for others. It's akin to playing a roulette game where the chances are bigger than previously.

what is good news? During pregnancy, especially in the second and third trimesters, many women report a reduction in the frequency and intensity of their migraines. The hormonal changes and increased blood flow that take place during pregnancy are typically attributed to this shift. However, for some unlucky individuals, pregnancy may either start a migraine or intensify an already existing one, especially in the first trimester.

EFFICACY OF PREVENTION

An active approach is essential to manage migraines during pregnancy. The key is to prevent. The following are some key techniques to help you prevent migraines:

Identify Triggers: Keep a careful lookout for probable migraine triggers. Some foods, stress, lack of sleep, and even seasonal changes are regular culprits. It could be highly good to maintain a migraine diary to spot patterns and avoid triggers.

Dehydration: Migraines can originate from dehydration. To stay hydrated, drink lots of water throughout the day. As a continuing reminder, bring a refillable water bottle with you.

Regular Meals: Skipping meals may result in low blood sugar, another migraine trigger. To maintain your blood sugar levels steady, make sure you consume regular, well-balanced meals.

Make Sleep A Priority And Build A Regular Sleep Schedule: A body that receives adequate sleep is less prone to migraines.

Reducing Stress Is Vital As Pregnancy Itself May Be Stressful: Use relaxation techniques like yoga, meditation, or deep breathing.

Consult Your Healthcare practitioner: Share any details about your migraines with your healthcare practitioner. They can aid you in discovering safe therapy solutions that are appropriate to your unique condition.

TREATMENT CONUNDRUM

The issue gets more problematic when it comes to controlling migraines during pregnancy. The majority of expecting moms opt to avoid using medicines, especially in the first trimester when the baby's organs are still forming. However, there are specific cases in which the risks of untreated migraines may be higher than those of certain remedies. A lengthy talk with your healthcare practitioner is important as it's a delicate balance.

There Are, However, Non-pharmacological Ways That May Give Relief:

- Applying a cold compress to your neck or forehead during a migraine episode could help minimize pain.
- As was previously noted, calming approaches like deep breathing and meditation may be beneficial pain treatment strategies.
- Biofeedback: This mind-body therapy assists in managing biological processes, such as muscle tension, that produce pain.
-

- Physical treatment: Physical therapy, as well as gentle neck and shoulder massages, may assist in minimizing the intensity and frequency of migraine episodes.
- Acupuncture: Some pregnant women find comfort in acupuncture, a traditional Chinese medicine treatment that involves placing small needles into particular body places.

Never undertake a new treatment or therapy without first visiting your healthcare practitioner.

As a consequence,
Pregnancy-related migraine care is a tough path, but it is one that may be successfully traversed with caution, knowledge, and the necessary support. Although there may be some rainy days, bear in mind that there will be brilliant skies in the future. You may enhance your chances of enjoying a more enjoyable and migraine-free pregnancy by

understanding triggers, practicing preventive strategies, and discussing with your doctor. You can accomplish this.

CAN MIGRAINES HAVE AN IMPACT ON SEXUAL HEALTH?

Imagine being in the mood for some alone time with your spouse when a debilitating migraine suddenly comes at your door. It's bothersome, isn't it? Although migraines are renowned for turning even the simplest delights into terrible ordeals, can they actually impair your sexual health? The answer is, unexpectedly, yes.

It is true that migraines, those unwelcome intruders in our heads, may influence our sexual lives. The connection between the two is a fascinating but frequently misinterpreted topic. In this inquiry, we explore the interesting relationship between sexual health and migraines, demonstrating how these two seemingly unrelated parts of life may interact in unanticipated ways.

THE SECRET ROUTES OF THE BRAIN
We need to grasp a basic idea: the brain's intricate networks -- in order to realize how migraines could impair our sexual health. Migraines are sophisticated neurological processes, not only headaches. Blood vessels in the brain tighten and then expand during a migraine attack, resulting in intense pain that is sometimes accompanied by additional symptoms like nausea and light sensitivity. These vascular alterations may start off a series of events in the brain that affect brain chemistry and perception.

The brain is responsible for a substantial percentage of sexual desire and response. The limbic system of the brain, which is in control of emotions and pleasure, is vital to the sexual experience. A migraine may accidentally change sexual desire and arousal when it interferes with the brain's typical functioning. As the pain and suffering become overriding distractions during a migraine episode, individuals may find themselves less receptive to connection.

CHANGES IN HORMONES

Your libido isn't helped by the hormonal ups and downs that occur during a migraine. It is commonly known that migraines impact oestrogen in particular. Hormonal fluctuations are typically associated with migraines in women, especially during the menstrual cycle.

Prior to menstruation, oestrogen levels fall, which in some individuals could result in migraines. Additional adverse effects of this hormonal imbalance include mood swings and a loss in sex drive. Therefore, a migraine may decrease your desire because it creates hormonal instability in addition to the physical anguish it brings.

THE FUNCTION OF MEDICINE

The utilization of medications are regularly used to regulate migraines, and here is where the narrative gets even more intriguing.

The unfavorable effects of various migraine therapies could have an influence on sexual health. For instance, as a side effect, some drugs may produce sexual dysfunction or diminished libido. When it comes to intimacy, this mix of migraines and their cures could make you feel as if you're in the center of a physical and emotional storm.

COMMUNICATION IS ESSENTIAL

Even if migraines may pose challenges to having a healthy sex life, there is good news: conversation may help narrow the gap. It may be highly good to have candid talks with your spouse about your experiences with migraines, their causes, and how they influence your sexual health. Navigating this perilous terrain with your partner's aid and understanding may be a game changer.

LOOKING FOR ASSISTANCE

You must receive professional care if migraines are continuously harming your sexual function and overall quality of life. Techniques for controlling migraines may lower the frequency and severity of attacks, which may gradually enhance your sexual health.

In summary, migraines are intricate neurological events that may impair a range of components of our lives, including our sexual health. They are more than merely bad headaches. The first step to effectively treating these concerns is to appreciate the relationship between migraines and sexual health.

You may aim towards having a healthy and enjoyable sex life even in the face of these terrible intruders in your mind by treating the physical and emotional components of migraines, seeking correct medical treatment, and preserving open communication with your partner.

PREVENTION

Can migraine headaches be prevented?
There is no cure for migraine headaches, but you can take an active part in managing them, maybe lowering how frequently you have them and potentially limiting how severe they are by following these tips:

- Keep a migraine journal. Take notes about any meals and other triggers that you believe may have led you to acquire a migraine. Make modifications in your diet and avoid such triggers as much as possible.
- Get a prescription for CGRP monoclonal antibodies. This injection was made particularly to aid in treating migraines.
- Get seven to nine hours of sleep a night.

- Eat at regular intervals. Don't miss meals. Drink lots of water.
- Exercise frequently and keep a healthy weight.
- Learn ways to manage stress such as meditation, yoga, relaxation training, or mindful breathing.
- Take drugs as advised by your healthcare practitioner. Preventative treatments include antidepressants, anti-seizure pharmaceuticals, calcitonin gene-related peptides, medicines that decrease blood pressure, and Botox injections. You could be administered timolol, amitriptyline, topiramate, and divalproex sodium. Notice that some of the same treatments that might help you manage a migraine may also help avoid one.
- Talk to your healthcare practitioner about hormone treatment if your migraines are suspected to be connected to your menstrual cycle.

- Consider attempting a transcutaneous supraorbital nerve stimulation device. This battery-powered electrical stimulator device is authorized by the Food and Drug Administration to prevent migraines. The gadget, worn like a headband or on your arm, generates electrical charges. The charge stimulates the nerve that transmits part of the pain experienced in migraine headaches. (The gadget may not be covered by your health insurance.)

- Get treatment with a professional for assistance regulating your stress. Ask your healthcare physician for a referral.

OUTLOOK / PROGNOSIS

What Is The Prognosis (outlook) For Patients With Migraines?

Migraines are unique to each person. Likewise, how migraines are controlled is also distinct. The greatest results are typically obtained by understanding and avoiding personal migraine triggers, managing symptoms, exercising preventative strategies, following the advice of your healthcare practitioner, and reporting any noteworthy changes as soon as they occur.

IS THERE A CURE FOR MIGRAINES?

Although there isn't a cure, there are therapies that may help you manage the symptoms.

HOW LONG WILL I HAVE MIGRAINE HEADACHES?

You may get migraine headaches for the rest of your life. If your migraines are triggered by your menstruation, you may cease suffering them when menopause begins.

QUESTIONS PEOPLE WITH MIGRAINES CAN ASK THEIR HEALTHCARE PROVIDER

- What's the specific reason for my migraines?
- Do migraines occur in various forms, and if so, which sort do I have?
- What often triggers migraines in me?
- How can I find out what causes my specific migraines?
- What adjustments can I make to my way of life to help prevent migraines?
- Should I make any dietary alterations to minimize the frequency of my migraines?
- Could my migraines be brought on by hormonal factors?
- How can I regulate my stress? What role does stress play in my migraines?
- Are there any vitamins or supplements that could assist in avoiding migraines?
- What migraine therapies are available, and how do they function?
- Should I be worried about any probable migraine medicine side effects?

- How can I know whether I should treat my migraines with over-the-counter medicines or prescription drugs?
- Do you have any recommendations for migraine cures that aren't drugs?
- Can you detail the pros and downsides of using triptans to cure migraines?
- Are there any fresh or cutting-edge migraine treatments I should be aware of?
- How can I build a customized migraine treatment strategy?
- How should a migraine diary be maintained, and why is it crucial?
- Are there any complementary or alternative treatments, such as acupuncture or biofeedback, that might aid with my migraines?
- Should I consider about getting Botox injections to prevent migraines, and how does it work?

- Can you explain "medication overuse headache" and let me know how to avoid it?
- What role does aura play in migraines, and how is it treated?
- Are there any special warning signals or indications that I should watch out for during a migraine attack so I can receive immediate medical help?
- What is the usual length of a migraine episode, and when should I be concerned if it lasts longer?
- Which emergency medicine do you advise I keep on hand in case I suffer a severe migraine attack?
- What should I do if my present course of treatment isn't working?
- Do menstrual migraines have any prevention measures?
- How frequently should I check in with you to evaluate how my migraine therapy is going?

- Are there any migraine-related clinical trials or research studies for which I may be qualified?
- Can you recommend any websites or support groups for folks who suffer from migraines?
- What probable long-term repercussions may repeated migraines have?
- Could another underlying medical problem be causing my migraines?
- Is there any concrete evidence that my migraines are increasing worse or occurring more frequently?
- How can I safely manage migraines while I'm expecting or nursing?
- Can you discuss the hazards of lengthy or recurrent use of medications for migraines?
- Are there any measures I should take to decrease migraine triggers when I travel?

- How can I notify my employer about my migraine condition and ask for any required accommodations?
- Can you give suggestions on how to manage migraines in youngsters or teenagers?
- Are there any concerns with living with chronic migraines that relate to mental health?
- What measures can I take to control my migraines and maintain a healthy lifestyle?
- Can you suggest a headache specialist or neurologist for additional testing and, if necessary, treatment?

CHAPTER 2

<u>THE MIGRAINE PUZZLE: Unveiling the Myths and Embracing the Facts</u>

In the winding paths of human experience, there are conditions that are shrouded in mystery and have been subject to numerous misconceptions and myths throughout the ages. Migraines, with their debilitating and enigmatic nature, are one such phenomenon.

They are not just headaches, but complex neurological events that have been a part of the human psyche since ancient times. In this chapter, we will explore the intricate maze of myths and facts that surround migraines, in an effort to dispel the shadows of ignorance and to embrace the illuminating truths that lie within.

Imagine a world where pain is a relentless force, capable of distorting reality, blurring the edges of perception, and leaving those who experience it in a state of constant fear. Migraines have been present in the annals of history, appearing in the earliest medical texts of antiquity, where they were often mistaken for supernatural afflictions.

Ancient civilizations, in their attempt to understand and interpret these agonizing events, created stories of divine displeasure or malevolent spirits as the cause, leaving generations to grapple with the burden of guilt and superstition.

Throughout the ages, myths about migraines have been pervasive in the collective consciousness, from the Greeks, who believed they were a punishment from the gods, to medieval Europe, where they were thought to be the result of demonic possession. In every corner of the globe, cultures developed their own narratives to explain this tormenting phenomenon, often casting blame upon the afflicted or seeking refuge in mysticism and magic. However, as humanity evolved and science advanced, it became increasingly evident that migraines were not the result of otherworldly forces, but had roots deeply entwined in the intricate circuitry of the human brain.

The myths surrounding migraines still exist today, perpetuated by misinformation, misunderstanding, and the enduring aura of mystique that surrounds this condition. Misconceptions that dismiss migraines as mere headaches, trivializing the profound suffering they inflict, are alarmingly common. Some still attribute these excruciating episodes to a weak constitution, overindulgence, or emotional instability, perpetuating stigmas that have plagued migraineurs for centuries.

However, as the light of modern science shines through the darkness of ignorance, a clearer understanding of migraines is emerging. With each new discovery, we move closer to unraveling the intricate web of factors that trigger these neurological storms. We now know that genetics, environmental factors, and an intricate interplay of neurochemicals are at the heart of migraines. Neuroimaging techniques have allowed us to witness the turmoil within the brain during an attack, shedding light on the physiological mechanisms that underlie this enigmatic condition.

In this chapter, we will embark on a journey of enlightenment, striving to differentiate between the myths and the realities that surround migraines. We will explore the historical, cultural, and scientific dimensions of this condition, dispelling misconceptions while embracing the wisdom that emerges from the ongoing quest for knowledge. Together, we will delve into the labyrinth of migraines, armed with facts, compassion, and a fervent desire to liberate those who suffer from the shadows of myth, offering a beacon of hope amidst the darkness of misunderstanding.

MYTH: Migraines are essentially acute headaches.
FACT: Migraines are a neurological disorder with diverse symptoms, generally accompanied by a pounding headache. They may include nausea, vomiting, and sensitivity to light and sound.

MYTH: Migraines are usually provoked by stress.
FACT: While stress may be a cause, migraines can also be induced by hormone changes, specific foods, weather, and other things.

MYTH: Only adults get migraines.
FACT: Migraines may afflict individuals of all ages, including children.

MYTH: You can cure a migraine with over-the-counter medicines.

FACT: Over-the-counter drugs may help reduce symptoms, but they do not cure migraines. Prescription drugs are typically required for successful therapy.

MYTH: Migraines are only an excuse to get out of work or social gatherings.

FACT: Migraines are a real medical ailment that may be very debilitating. People with migraines typically cannot function properly during an episode.

MYTH: Migraines are not inherited.

FACT: Genetics may have a crucial impact on the development of migraines. If one or both parents experience migraines, you are at a greater risk.

MYTH: You may prevent migraines by avoiding all triggers.

FACT: While trigger avoidance may assist, it's not always feasible to avoid all triggers, and certain triggers are still not fully understood.

MYTH: Migraines are a woman's concern.
FACT: Migraines are more frequent in women, although they afflict males as well.

MYTH: Migraines are merely a severe headache, and you can fight it out.
FACT: Migraines may be incredibly painful and debilitating, making it hard to go on with usual activities.

MYTH: Migraines just affect your head.
FACT: Migraines may have a broad variety of symptoms, including visual problems, numbness or tingling in the body, and gastrointestinal troubles.

MYTH: Migraines are usually preceded by an aura.
FACT: While some migraines occur with an aura (visual disturbances), many do not.

MYTH: You can't exercise if you get migraines.

FACT: Regular exercise may really help lessen the frequency and intensity of migraines for some individuals.

MYTH: Migraines are triggered by eating chocolate.

FACT: While chocolate may provoke migraines in some folks, it's not a universal trigger.

MYTH: Migraines are psychological.

FACT: Migraines have a neurological foundation and are not solely psychological.

MYTH: You can outgrow migraines.

FACT: Migraines may endure throughout a person's life, but they may become less common as you become older.

MYTH: Migraines are all the same.

FACT: There are numerous forms of migraines, including migraines with aura, migraines without aura, chronic migraines, and more, each with distinct features.

MYTH: Migraines are always provoked by eating.
FACT: Food triggers are only one of several possible migraine triggers, and they differ from person to person.

MYTH: You can't work with a migraine.
FACT: Some individuals can function to some degree during a migraine episode, while others are entirely paralyzed.

MYTH: Migraines are usually preceded by a warning sign.
FACT: While some migraines begin with a warning sign or aura, others might hit unexpectedly.

MYTH: Migraines are solely a vascular disease.

FACT: Migraines involve complicated brain processes, and their precise etiology is still not entirely known.

MYTH: You can't experience more than one migraine in a day.
FACT: Some patients get many headaches in a single day, termed as a migraine attack or condition migrainosus.

MYTH: You can't have a migraine if you've never experienced one before.
FACT: Migraines may occur at any time in your life, even if you've never had one before.

MYTH: Migraines are merely a minor annoyance.
FACT: Migraines may be very debilitating and impact a person's quality of life.

MYTH: You can tough it out without therapy.

FACT: Treatment is typically essential to ease the pain and other symptoms of migraines.

MYTH: Migraines are usually on one side of the head.

FACT: While many migraines are one-sided, they may also be bilateral, affecting both sides of the brain.

MYTH: All migraines are the same for everyone.

FACT: Migraines differ from person to person, both in terms of symptoms and causes.

MYTH: Migraines are caused by sinus issues.

FACT: Sinus difficulties may induce headache-like symptoms, but they are not the same as migraines.

MYTH: Migraines only last a few hours.

FACT: Migraines may persist for a few hours to many days, with varied degrees of severity.

MYTH: Migraines are usually followed by vomiting.
FACT: Nausea and vomiting are frequent migraine symptoms but not present in every instance.

MYTH: You can't suffer migraines during pregnancy.
FACT: Migraines may remain or even worsen during pregnancy, although treatment choices may be restricted owing to safety concerns.

MYTH: Migraines are only a reaction to stress.
FACT: While stress may provoke migraines, they are a complicated neurological disorder with several contributing components.

MYTH: Migraines are only an excuse for prescription drugs.

FACT: Prescription drugs for migraines are frequently essential for good relief and are not used as an excuse.

MYTH: Migraines are an indication of a brain tumor.

FACT: While it's necessary to rule out significant medical disorders, most migraines are not related with brain tumors.

MYTH: Migraines are caused by poor eating.

FACT: Diet may be a trigger for some individuals, but it's not the primary cause of migraines.

MYTH: Migraines are a consequence of poor sleep patterns.

FACT: Poor sleep may provoke migraines in certain people, but it's not the sole reason.

MYTH: Migraines are a sort of seizure.

FACT: Migraines and seizures are separate neurological diseases with different underlying processes.

MYTH: Migraines may be healed with surgery.

FACT: There is no medical cure for migraines, however, certain surgical treatments may help ease symptoms in select circumstances.

MYTH: Migraines are only a response to bright lighting.

FACT: While light sensitivity (photophobia) is a typical migraine symptom, it's not the sole cause.

MYTH: Migraines usually have a precise pattern or timetable.

FACT: Migraines may arise unexpectedly and may not follow a regular pattern.

MYTH: Migraines are only a consequence of overthinking.

FACT: Migraines are not caused by overthinking or psychological causes alone.

MYTH: Migraines are infectious.

FACT: Migraines are not infectious and cannot be passed from person to person.

MYTH: Migraines are an indication of poor willpower.

FACT: Migraines are a medical ailment and have nothing to do with willpower.

MYTH: Migraines are not a major health concern.

FACT: Migraines may have a substantial influence on a person's life and may lead to disability if not adequately controlled.

MYTH: Migraines usually start in infancy.

FACT: Migraines may occur at any age, even maturity.

MYTH: Migraines may be avoided by avoiding all triggers.
FACT: While trigger avoidance might assist, it's not always easy to recognize or avoid all triggers.

MYTH: Migraines are always provoked by drinking.
FACT: Alcohol may be a trigger for certain people, although not everyone with migraines is affected by it.

MYTH: Migraines are caused by excessive blood pressure.
FACT: While high blood pressure may contribute to many health complications, it's not a direct cause of migraines.

MYTH: Migraines are only a consequence of dehydration.
FACT: Dehydration may be a trigger for some individuals, but it's not the primary cause of migraines.

MYTH: Migraines are usually accompanied by auras.

FACT: Many migraines develop without any aura or warning signals.

MYTH: Migraines may be healed by a certain diet.

FACT: While dietary adjustments may help some people manage their migraines, there is no one-size-fits-all diet for migraine treatment.

MYTH: Migraines are caused by allergies.

FACT: Allergies may produce sinus headaches, which may be mistaken for migraines, but they are not the same.

MYTH: Migraines are only a consequence of lack of activity.

FACT: While regular exercise may help lessen the frequency and intensity of migraines, they are not primarily caused by a lack of physical activity.

MYTH: Migraines are usually accompanied by a visual aura.

FACT: Auras are simply one form of migraine, and many migraines do not include visual abnormalities as a symptom.

MYTH: Migraines are entirely in your mind.

FACT: Migraines include physical, neurological, and hereditary components and are not a result of imagination or psychological disorders.

MYTH: Migraines may be healed with a simple home treatment.

FACT: While certain home treatments may give relief for minor migraines, they are not a solution for the illness. Effective therapy typically involves medical intervention.

MYTH: Migraines are usually provoked by strong scents.

FACT: Strong fragrances might be a trigger for some individuals, although not all migraines are connected to smells.

MYTH: Migraines are usually accompanied by extreme nausea.
FACT: Nausea may be a symptom of migraines, however not everyone with migraines gets it.

MYTH: Migraines are only a consequence of allergies.
FACT: Allergies may produce sinus headaches, which may be mistaken for migraines, but they are not the same.

CHAPTER 3

<u>BEYOND PAINKILLERS:</u> <u>Exploring Alternatives</u>

INTRODUCTION TO COMPLEMENTARY AND ALTERNATIVE TREATMENTS(CAM) FOR MIGRAINES
- Definition and Overview
- Importance of Alternative Approaches

Picture this: you're going about your day, minding your own thing, when suddenly, a searing agony grabs your brain like a vice. Lights become your foes, and even the gentlest noises seem like a jackhammer in your brain. Welcome to the realm of migraines, where orthodox therapies often fall short, and that's when complementary and alternative remedies come into play.

Before we enter into the interesting area of alternative migraine cures, let's clear up some terminology. Complementary and alternative therapies (CAM) are healthcare approaches that operate beyond the sphere of mainstream medicine. They complement your usual therapies or give alternatives to them. Now, suppose you're on a treasure hunt, and conventional medicine is your trusty map, while CAM is the X designating the area where relief lives.

When it comes to migraines, CAM comprises a large diversity of therapies, each giving a distinct approach to alleviating migraine discomfort. These techniques may be roughly grouped into:

MIND-BODY METHODS: These methods harness the power of your mind to overcome migraines. Practices like meditation, biofeedback, and relaxation exercises help you achieve greater control over your body's reaction to pain.

HERBAL CURES AND SUPPLEMENTS: Nature has a variety of cures up its sleeve. Ginger, butterbur, and magnesium supplements are just a few examples of natural compounds that some feel might ease migraine symptoms.

ACUPUNCTURE: A therapy based on ancient Chinese medicine, acupuncture involves putting small needles into precise places on your body to regulate the flow of qi. This therapy seeks to ease migraine discomfort and lessen its frequency.

DIET AND LIFESTYLE CHANGES: What you eat and how you live may substantially affect your migraines. Eliminating trigger foods, keeping hydrated, and having a regular sleep pattern are all part of this CAM category.

PHYSICAL THERAPIES: Chiropractic adjustments and osteopathic manipulative treatment (OMT) concentrate on realigning your body's structures to reduce migraine symptoms.

ENERGY HEALING: Practices like Reiki and therapeutic touch involve channeling energy to facilitate physical and emotional healing. While the scientific foundation may be contested, many patients report decreased migraine severity and frequency following these sessions.

IMPORTANCE OF ALTERNATIVE APPROACHES FOR MANAGING MIGRAINES

Now, you may ask why anybody would seek these alternative techniques when mainstream medicine exists. Well, the answer lies in the multidimensional character of migraines and the reality that what works for one individual may not work for another.

PERSONALIZATION: Migraines are not one-size-fits-all. They vary in severity, frequency, and triggers from person to person. CAM therapies can allow for a more tailored approach, adapting cures to individual requirements.

REDUCING MEDICATION DEPENDENCY: Conventional migraine treatments may often have negative effects or become less effective over time. CAM provides alternate routes to relief, possibly lowering the need for long-term pharmaceutical usage.

HOLISTIC WELL-BEING: CAM frequently focuses on treating the full individual rather than just the symptoms. This comprehensive approach may enhance total well-being, treating not just physical pain but also the emotional and psychological elements of migraines.

EMPOWERMENT: Engaging in CAM therapies encourages people to take an active role in controlling their migraines. It increases self-awareness and the development of abilities to deal with suffering.

In conclusion, complementary and alternative therapies for migraines bring up a world of options outside the constraints of standard therapy. While not a definite solution, they provide hope, personalization, and empowerment to individuals seeking respite from the devastating hold of migraines. So, if you're on a journey for pain treatment, don't be scared to explore the unexplored region of CAM — you could just uncover the treasure trove of relief you've been seeking.

COMMON HERBAL REMEDIES
FEVERFEW
- Dosage and Usage
- Effectiveness and Research
BUTTERBUR
- Dosage and Usage

- Effectiveness and Research
PEPPERMINT OIL
- Dosage and Usage
- Effectiveness and Research

While traditional medicine provides many treatments, some individuals seek comfort in natural therapies. In this investigation of typical herbal therapies for migraines, we will dive into the exciting world of feverfew, butterbur, and peppermint oil.

FEVERFEW AS A NATURAL REMEDY FOR MIGRAINES

DOSAGE AND USAGE OF FEVERFEW FOR MIGRAINES

Feverfew, a flowering plant with a name that emphasizes its fever-reducing effects, has been used for generations as a natural cure for migraines. Typically, feverfew is ingested in capsule form, with a suggested dose ranging from 50 to 150 mg daily. You may also make it into a tea or chew on the raw leaves, though the latter can be extremely harsh.

EFFECTIVENESS AND RESEARCH ON FEVERFEW FOR MIGRAINES

The efficacy of feverfew in avoiding migraines has attracted attention from the scientific community. Multiple studies have demonstrated that frequent use of feverfew may lower the frequency and severity of migraine episodes. The herb is thought to function by lowering inflammation and constriction of blood vessels in the brain, both of which are essential contributors to migraine onset.

However, it's vital to remember that feverfew doesn't bring quick relief. It may take many weeks of constant usage to notice effects. As with any herbal medicine, it's advisable to contact a healthcare expert before adding feverfew to your migraine management regimen.

BUTTERBUR

DOSAGE AND USAGE OF BUTTERBUR FOR MIGRAINES

Butterbur, another herbal rival in the war against migraines, is extracted from the root of the butterbur plant. Typically available in pill or tablet form, the suggested dose for butterbur extract is roughly 75 mg twice a day. Unlike feverfew, taking fresh butterbur leaves is not suggested owing to possibly hazardous chemicals.

EFFECTIVENESS & RESEARCH ON BUTTERBUR FOR MIGRAINES

Butterbur has proved its mettle in clinical studies. Studies show that it may greatly lower the frequency and severity of migraine episodes when taken regularly. Butterbur's mode of action includes inhibiting the dilatation of blood arteries in the brain, hence thwarting one of the key causes of migraines.

One major concern while using Butterbur is verifying that the product is labeled "PA-free." This implies that it does not contain pyrrolizidine alkaloids, which may be hazardous to the liver. Consult a healthcare expert before beginning any butterbur program to confirm it's safe for you.

PEPPERMINT OIL AS A NATURAL REMEDY FOR MIGRAINES

DOSAGE AND USAGE OF PEPPERMINT OIL FOR MIGRAINES

Peppermint oil, with its pleasant scent, has gained favor as a natural cure for migraines. It's often administered topically, diluted with a carrier oil like coconut oil, to the temples and forehead. A few drops of peppermint oil may also be put in a bowl of hot water for inhalation.

EFFECTIVENESS AND RESEARCH ON PEPPERMINT OIL FOR MIGRAINES

Research on peppermint oil's usefulness for migraines is encouraging, but rather restricted. The cooling feeling offered by peppermint oil may help relax stiff muscles in the head and neck, thereby relieving migraine-related discomfort.

One research indicated that breathing peppermint oil lessened the severity of headaches. However, a more detailed study is required to confirm its effectiveness clearly. As with any essential oil, it's necessary to dilute peppermint oil appropriately and do a patch test to check for skin sensitivity.

In conclusion, three herbal remedies—feverfew, butterbur, and peppermint oil—offer possible assistance for migraine patients. While they may not work for everyone, their natural qualities make them worth considering as supplementary therapies. Remember, always visit a healthcare practitioner before going on any herbal treatment journey, and maintain a migraine journal to document your improvement. Relief from migraines may be closer than you believe, nestled inside the embrace of nature's healing herbs.

LESSER-KNOWN HERBAL REMEDIES

GINGER
- Dosage and Usage
- Effectiveness and Research

LAVENDER OIL
- Dosage and Usage
- Effectiveness and Research

WILLOW BARK
- Dosage and Usage
- Effectiveness and Research

In this examination of lesser-known herbal medicines, we dive into the calming effects of ginger, the scented appeal of lavender oil, and the bark of the willow tree, all of which have shown promise in the struggle against migraines.

GINGER AS A HERBAL REMEDY FOR MIGRAINES

DOSAGE AND USAGE OF GINGER FOR MIGRAINES

Ginger, a spicy root frequently found in kitchens worldwide, has a long history of therapeutic usage. To leverage its migraine-fighting power, you may prepare ginger in numerous forms:

- Ginger Tea: Slice or grate fresh ginger root (approximately 1-2 tablespoons), simmer it in boiling water for 5-10 minutes, and enjoy a nice cup of ginger tea. Add honey for sweetness, if preferred.
- Ginger Capsules: Ginger supplements are available in pill form. Follow the

indicated dose on the box, often about 250-500 mg.

- Ginger Oil: Dilute a few drops of ginger essential oil with a carrier oil (like coconut oil) and massage your temples and neck for comfort.

EFFECTIVENESS AND RESEARCH OF GINGER FOR MIGRAINES

Ginger's promise for migraine treatment resides in its anti-inflammatory and pain-relieving qualities. Some studies show that ginger may help lower the severity and frequency of migraines when taken frequently. However, individual reactions might differ, and additional study is required to confirm its usefulness definitely.

LAVENDER OIL AS A NATURAL REMEDY FOR MIGRAINES

DOSAGE AND USAGE OF LAVENDER OIL FOR MIGRAINES

Lavender, renowned for its appealing perfume, also possesses medicinal qualities that help ease migraine symptoms:

- Aromatherapy: Add a few drops of lavender essential oil to a basin of boiling hot water. Inhale the calming vapor for 15-20 minutes.
- Lavender Oil Topical Application: Dilute lavender essential oil with a carrier oil, such as almond or jojoba oil, and gently massage your temples and neck.

EFFECTIVENESS AND RESEARCH ON LAVENDER OIL FOR MIGRAINES

Lavender oil's relaxing aroma may help relieve stress and anxiety, which frequent migraine causes. Several studies have studied its potential in controlling migraines, indicating that inhaling lavender oil may lead to a considerable decrease in headache intensity and duration. While it may not work for everyone, it gives a natural, pleasant choice for relief.

WILLOW BARK AS A HERBAL REMEDY FOR MIGRAINES

DOSAGE AND USAGE OF WILLOW BARK FOR MIGRAINES

Willow bark, a natural source of salicin, which is comparable to aspirin, has been used for generations to reduce pain, especially migraines:

- Willow Bark Tea: Steep one to two tablespoons of dried willow bark in boiling water for around 10-15 minutes and consume it as a tea. This strategy is comparable to utilizing aspirin for headache relief.
- Willow Bark Extract: Willow bark extracts are available in numerous forms, including capsules and

tinctures. Follow the suggested dose on the product packaging.

EFFECTIVENESS & RESEARCH OF WILLOW BARK FOR MIGRAINES

Willow bark's possible usefulness for migraines may be linked to its anti-inflammatory and pain-relieving qualities. Some studies show that it may offer relief from headache symptoms, but additional study is essential to validate its efficacy and safety as a long-term migraine cure.

In the area of migraine care, lesser-known herbal therapies like ginger, lavender oil, and willow bark offer fascinating possibilities. While they may not work for everyone, they give natural options that are worth trying alongside orthodox therapies. Always contact a healthcare practitioner before beginning any new migraine treatment regimen to confirm it's safe and suitable for your unique situation.

HERBAL TEAS AND INFUSIONS
Chamomile Tea
- Dosage and Usage
- Effectiveness and Research
Valerian Root Tea
- Dosage and Usage
- Effectiveness and Research

Imagine a relaxing, scented cup of herbal tea in your hands, slowly alleviating the hammering in your brain, and bringing refuge from the unyielding grip of a migraine. This isn't just a lovely fantasy; it's a realistic reality when you explore the world of herbal mixes and recipes for migraine treatment.

Nature has gifted us with an assortment of strong herbs, each with distinct traits that, when combined, generate synergistic effects capable of reducing migraine symptoms. In this inquiry, we'll dig into the relaxing realm of herbal teas and their possible advantages for migraines.

CHAMOMILE TEA FOR MIGRAINES

DOSAGE AND USAGE OF CHAMOMILE TEA FOR MIGRAINES:
Chamomile tea, made from the dried flowers of the chamomile plant, is well-known for its relaxing and anti-inflammatory qualities. To harness its potential advantages for migraines, take these easy steps:

- Select Quality Ingredients: Start with high-quality chamomile tea bags or dried chamomile flowers. Organic choices are recommended to guarantee purity.
- Steeping Process: Boil water and let it cool slightly to around 200°F (93°C). Pour it over your chamomile tea bag or a spoonful of dried chamomile flowers in a cup.
- Steep Time: Allow the tea to steep for approximately 5 minutes, or alter the

steeping time according to your desire for flavor and strength.

- Sweeten or Not: While optional, you may add honey or lemon to improve the flavor. However, it's vital to prevent excessive sweetening, since sugar might possibly provoke migraines in certain persons.

EFFECTIVENESS AND RESEARCH OF CHAMOMILE TEA FOR MIGRAINES:

Chamomile tea's potential benefit against migraines is founded in its anti-inflammatory and relaxing effects. The tea includes chemicals including chamazulene and apigenin, which display anti-inflammatory and muscle-relaxant actions, possibly reducing migraine-related stress.

Research on chamomile tea's migraine-relieving qualities is ongoing but encouraging. Some studies have shown that the tea may help lessen the frequency and severity of migraines. However, individual reactions may vary, and it's vital to contact with a healthcare practitioner before taking chamomile tea as a migraine cure, particularly if you have any allergies or sensitivities.

VALERIAN ROOT TEA FOR MIGRAINES

DOSAGE AND USAGE OF VALERIAN ROOT TEA FOR MIGRAINES:
Valerian root tea is recognized for its relaxing and sedative qualities. To examine its possible advantages for migraine treatment, here's a basic guide:

- Choose the Right Ingredients: Opt for high-quality valerian root tea bags or valerian root extract.
- Brewing Process: Boil water and let it cool somewhat to roughly 212°F (100°C). Place a valerian root tea bag

or pour a suggested quantity of valerian root extract into your cup.

- Steeping Time: Allow the tea to steep for about 5-10 minutes. Adjust the steeping time according to your desire for flavor and intensity.
- Optional Enhancements: While not essential, you may add a bit of honey or a slice of lemon to improve the flavor.

EFFECTIVENESS AND RESEARCH OF VALERIAN ROOT TEA FOR MIGRAINES:

Valerian root has been used for generations as a cure for anxiety and sleeplessness, mostly owing to its relaxing qualities. While there isn't an abundance of studies explicitly focused on valerian root tea for migraines, its possible benefits may be connected to its ability to relieve tension and induce relaxation.

It's crucial to remember that valerian root may have sedative effects, therefore it's advised to drink it in a safe setting and avoid activities that demand awareness, such as driving, after taking valerian root tea.

In conclusion, herbal teas like chamomile and valerian root provide possible assistance for migraine patients via their relaxing and anti-inflammatory characteristics.

While these natural therapies might be effective, it's vital to check with a healthcare practitioner before adopting them into your migraine management strategy, particularly if you have any underlying health concerns or are using drugs. With the appropriate instruction, herbal teas may give a calming way to a migraine-free day.

COMBINING HERBS FOR MIGRAINE RELIEF
- **Herbal Blends and Recipes**
- **Synergistic Effects**

Imagine a life free from the throbbing pain of a migraine, where you can appreciate every moment without the lurking dread of an oncoming headache. For some who fight migraines, this image can seem like a faraway dream.

However, nature has a way of delivering consolation via plants. Welcome to the realm of mixing herbs for migraine treatment, where the power of nature's remedies may work in harmony to reduce your pain.

HERBAL BLENDS AND RECIPES FOR MIGRAINES

FEVERFEW AND BUTTERBUR DUO:
Feverfew and butterbur are herbal superstars when it comes to migraine treatment. Feverfew, with its anti-inflammatory characteristics, helps to lower the severity and frequency of migraines.

On the other hand, butterbur has been demonstrated to relax blood vessels and decrease spasms, which are typically causes of migraines. Together, they constitute a formidable combination.

RECIPE: Create a tincture by blending dried feverfew and butterbur root in equal portions. Take a dropperful daily to prevent migraines or increase the dosage during an attack for rapid relief.

LAVENDER AND PEPPERMINT SYMPHONY:

Lavender, renowned for its relaxing scent, may help reduce stress-induced migraines. Peppermint, with its calming and anti-inflammatory characteristics, compliments lavender well. When mixed, these herbs form a balanced mixture that treats both the physical and emotional elements of migraines.

RECIPE: Make a calming tea by infusing dried lavender flowers and peppermint leaves. Sip on this aromatic tea during the early stages of a migraine to lessen discomfort and soothe your thoughts.

GINGER AND TURMERIC ELIXIR:
Ginger and turmeric, two culinary classics, provide a potent pair for migraine treatment. Ginger's anti-inflammatory characteristics may help lessen pain and nausea associated with migraines, while turmeric gives a natural boost to your body's anti-inflammatory reactions.

RECIPE: Combine fresh ginger root slices and turmeric powder with boiling water. Add honey for a touch of sweetness and drink this warming elixir to alleviate migraine agony.

SYNERGISTIC EFFECTS OF COMBINING HERBS FOR MIGRAINE RELIEF

The magic of mixing herbs for migraine treatment resides in the notion of synergy. It's like forming a team of superheroes, where each herb brings its particular abilities to the table, increasing the entire impact.

- Enhanced Efficacy: When herbs operate together, they might give more substantial relief than when administered singly. For example, the anti-inflammatory effects of ginger and turmeric together may attack many routes of migraine development concurrently.
- Balanced Effects: Some herbs may cause side effects when ingested in big numbers. However, when mixed wisely, they may counteract each other, minimizing the chance of unwanted responses. This harmony might make your herbal medicine safer and more pleasurable.

- Comprehensive Relief: Migraines are complicated, including many causes and symptoms. Combining herbs helps you to attack many components of the ailment, such as pain, nausea, and stress, all at once. This holistic strategy may considerably enhance your overall quality of life.

In conclusion, the world of herbal mixes and recipes for migraine treatment is a treasure trove waiting to be discovered. By utilizing the synergistic benefits of mixing herbs, you may unleash the power of nature to ease your migraine agony. Embrace these natural cures, and take a step closer to a life where migraines no longer dominate your everyday lives.

SAFETY PRECAUTIONS AND SIDE EFFECTS

- Interactions with Medications
- Allergies and Sensitivities

Herbal therapies for migraines have gained popularity owing to their natural origins and probable efficiency. However, the route to migraine treatment using herbs must be traversed with prudence.

In this research, we look into the safety precautions and possible side effects of herbal medicines for migraines, finding the complicated web of interactions with drugs, as well as the role allergies and sensitivities play in this natural approach to controlling migraines.

SAFETY PRECAUTIONS: NAVIGATING THE NATURAL TERRAIN

- Speak With A Healthcare Professional: Before going on any herbal treatment journey, speak with a healthcare practitioner. They may help you decide whether herbal remedies are suited for your individual illness, including any underlying health conditions or drugs you may be taking.

- Research and Source Authentic Products: Not all herbal treatments are made equal. assure you acquire herbs from trusted suppliers to prevent contamination and assure the purity and potency of the product.
- Dosage Awareness: Herbal treatments should be taken in the proper dosage. Excessive use may lead to harmful consequences, while minimal amounts may not give relief. Always follow the suggested doses on product labels or as instructed by your healthcare practitioner.
- Gradual Introduction: When attempting a new herbal cure, incorporate it gradually into your regimen to monitor any possible side effects or allergic responses.

SIDE EFFECTS: NAVIGATING THE BUMPS ON THE HERBAL ROAD

- Gastrointestinal Upsets: Some herbal medicines might irritate the stomach lining, resulting in nausea, vomiting, or diarrhea. Ginger and peppermint, renowned for their digestive characteristics, help ease these sensations.
- Blood Pressure Oscillations: Certain herbs, such as feverfew and butterbur, have been associated with oscillations in blood pressure. Monitoring your blood pressure periodically while taking these medicines is vital.
- Liver And Kidney Concerns: Long-term usage of certain herbs, including butterbur, may have ramifications for liver health. Regular liver function tests are suggested in such circumstances.

INTERACTIONS WITH MEDICATIONS: THE HERB-DRUG TANGO

- Blood Thinners: Some herbal treatments like feverfew and ginkgo biloba contain blood-thinning qualities. When used with blood-thinning drugs like warfarin, it may increase the risk of bleeding.

- Antidepressants: St. John's Wort, often used for migraines, might interact with antidepressant drugs, thereby lowering its efficacy.
- Blood Pressure Medications: Herbs like valerian may drop blood pressure, which might be troublesome if you're currently using medicine to manage blood pressure.
- Migraine drugs: Combining herbal treatments with migraine drugs might result in unanticipated reactions. Always notify your healthcare professional about any therapies and drugs you're consuming.

ALLERGIES AND SENSITIVITIES: UNMASKING HIDDEN TRIGGERS

- Individual Variability: Just like with food allergies, individuals might be sensitive or allergic to various plants. Common allergies in herbal treatments include chamomile, echinacea, and lavender. Start with a small dose and monitor for any adverse responses such as skin rashes or trouble breathing.

- Cross-Allergies: If you have known allergies to particular plants, be careful while utilizing herbal medicines produced from related plants, since cross-allergies might arise. For example, if you're sensitive to ragweed, you may also react to chamomile.

In conclusion, the realm of herbal medicines for migraines provides a potential road to relief. However, it's vital to proceed cautiously, considering safety considerations, possible side effects, prescription combinations, and the risk of allergies. Consulting with a healthcare physician and keeping watchful about your body's reactions can help you traverse this natural terrain and maybe get the migraine relief you want while avoiding undesirable effects. Remember, nature's medicine is broad, but knowledge and prudence are your greatest guides.

LIFESTYLE CHANGES TO COMPLEMENT HERBAL REMEDIES
- Diet and Nutrition
- Stress Management Techniques
- Sleep Hygiene

While herbal medicines may bring relief, they're most successful when accompanied by lifestyle adjustments that support your search for migraine control. In this road towards a migraine-free life, three main pillars play a critical role: Diet and Nutrition, Stress Management Techniques, and Sleep Hygiene. Together, they offer a comprehensive strategy that not only supports natural medicines but also allows you to retake control over your life. Let's go on this interesting and easy-to-understand investigation of these lifestyle modifications that may make a world of difference in your migraine struggle.

DIET & NUTRITION FOR MIGRAINES:
Imagine your body as a highly tuned machine, and the fuel it operates on substantially affects its performance. When it comes to controlling migraines, your food and nutrition choices may be a game-changer. Here's how you can make it work for you:

- Stay Hydrated: Dehydration may exacerbate migraines, so make water your closest friend. Aim for at least eight glasses of water a day to keep those headaches at bay.
- Identify Trigger Meals: Certain meals might behave as migraine triggers. Common causes include processed meals, caffeine, alcohol, aged cheeses, and artificial sweeteners. Keep a

record to discover your individual triggers and avoid them.

- Mindful Eating: Rushed meals might upset blood sugar levels and increase your vulnerability to migraines. Practice attentive eating by enjoying each meal, and keep regular eating patterns to balance blood sugar.
- Balanced Diet: Incorporate a balanced diet rich in fruits, vegetables, whole grains, lean meats, and healthy fats. Avoid abrupt food changes, since these might provoke headaches due to blood sugar swings.
- Magnesium and Riboflavin: Include foods high in magnesium (such as nuts and leafy greens) and riboflavin (found in dairy, lean meats, and green vegetables) in your diet, since these nutrients may help lessen migraine frequency.

STRESS MANAGEMENT TECHNIQUES FOR MIGRAINES:

Stress is like a quiet saboteur, lurking in the background, waiting to cause a migraine at the most inopportune moments. Here are stress management tactics to fight this unrelenting foe:

- awareness & Meditation: Cultivate awareness via meditation and deep breathing exercises. These strategies may help you remain present, decreasing anxiety and minimizing stress-induced migraines.
- Regular Exercise: Engaging in regular physical exercise generates endorphins, your body's natural stress fighters. Find a fitness program you love, whether it's yoga, swimming, or a simple daily stroll.
- Time Management: Effective time management helps reduce last-minute rushes and the resulting stress. Use calendars and to-do lists to keep organized and in control.

- Set Boundaries: Learn to say "no" when required. Overcommitting may lead to prolonged stress, which is a fertile environment for migraines.
- relaxing Techniques: Explore relaxing techniques such as progressive muscle relaxation, aromatherapy, or calming baths. These may help you relax and melt away tension.

SLEEP HYGIENE FOR MIGRAINES:
Sleep is your body's natural reset button, and maintaining proper sleep hygiene is vital for migraine control. Here's how you can increase your sleep quality:

- Consistent Sleep Schedule: Go to bed and wake up at the same time every day, including on weekends. Consistency supports your body's intrinsic clock.
- Create a Sleep-Inducing Environment: Make your bedroom a refuge for sleep.

Keep it cold, dark, and silent. Invest in a comfy mattress and pillows.

- Limit Screen Time: The blue light generated by screens might interfere with your sleep habits. Avoid screens at least one hour before sleep.
- Mind relaxing: Practice relaxing methods before bed. You might try reading a peaceful book, moderate stretching, or progressive muscular relaxation to ease into sleep.
- Caffeine and Alcohol: Limit caffeine and alcohol consumption, particularly in the evening. These drugs might interrupt your sleep pattern.

Incorporating these lifestyle modifications with natural medicines will enable you to restore control over your life and experience migraine-free days. Remember, consistency is crucial, and with time, these methods may become second nature, lessening the frequency and intensity of your migraines. So, go on this comprehensive road towards a migraine-free life, one step at a time, and appreciate the newfound freedom it gives.

MIND-BODY PRACTICES
- Yoga for Migraine Relief
- Meditation and Mindfulness

While drugs might help control symptoms, there's a holistic alternative that's been gaining attention and offering comfort to many sufferers: mind-body activities. These disciplines, including yoga, meditation, and mindfulness, provide a ray of hope for migraine treatment that surpasses the constraints of medicines. In this trip, we will dig into two of the most powerful mind-body practices: Yoga and Meditation, investigating how they may help you discover the secrets to a migraine-free life.

YOGA FOR MIGRAINE RELIEF:
Picture this: you're in a softly lit room, gentle music playing in the background, and you're flowing effortlessly through a

sequence of stances. This is the world of yoga, and it could well be your ticket to a life with fewer migraines. Here's how it works.

- Stress Reduction: One of the major migraine causes is stress. Yoga, with its gentle postures and concentration on deep breathing, is a natural stress-buster. As you flow through postures and focus on your breath, your body relaxes, and stress levels fall. This decrease in stress may dramatically lower the frequency and severity of your migraines.
- Improved Blood Flow: Yoga is all about balance, and doing it frequently may enhance your blood circulation. This improved blood flow guarantees that oxygen and nutrients reach your brain more effectively, minimizing the probability of migraine episodes.
- Release of Tension: Migraines generally arise from muscular tension in the neck and shoulders. Yoga's

stretching and relaxation practices may help relieve this tension, delivering instant relief and avoiding future headaches.

- Mind-Body Connection: Yoga isn't only about physical postures; it's about connecting your mind and body. With enhanced knowledge, you may identify migraine causes early and take preventive steps.
- Better Sleep: Poor sleep may be a migraine cause. Yoga's relaxing benefits help you sleep better, ensuring your body is well-rested and less vulnerable to migraine episodes.

MEDITATION AND MINDFULNESS FOR MIGRAINES:
Imagine a tranquil landscape inside your imagination, where cares dissolve away like morning mist. Meditation and mindfulness are your tools to create this inner serenity, and they have enormous promise for migraine control.

- Tension reduction and Relaxation: Similar to yoga, meditation, and mindfulness relieve tension and promote relaxation. By concentrating on your breath or a relaxing mantra, you may let go of the tension that commonly accompanies a migraine.
- Pain Perception: Migraines are severe, but your perception of that pain may be adjusted via meditation. By training your mind to accept pain, you may minimize the apparent intensity of migraines.
- Trigger Awareness: Mindfulness teaches you to be present in the moment, and to examine your thoughts, emotions, and bodily sensations without judgment. This heightened awareness may help you detect migraine triggers, whether they're connected to diet, environment, or stress.
- Coping Mechanisms: Meditation offers you mental skills to deal with

discomfort. Instead of panicking during a migraine episode, you may utilize meditation methods to keep calm and handle the pain more successfully.

- Preventive Benefits: Regular meditation and mindfulness practice may really lower the frequency and severity of migraines over time. By building mental resilience, you construct a fortress against future assaults.

In conclusion, the realm of mind-body activities provides a potential road towards migraine treatment. Yoga, with its stress-reducing, tension-releasing, and circulation-boosting effects, may considerably help your migraine treatment. Meanwhile, meditation and mindfulness allow you to shift your connection with pain and boost your capacity to detect and minimize triggers. So, take a step into this holistic world, where the mind and body work in unison to provide you with a life with fewer migraines and more moments of exquisite tranquility.

ACUPUNCTURE AND ACUPRESSURE
- How Acupuncture Works
- Pressure Points for Migraine Relief

Migraines may be nothing short of devastating, producing throbbing pain, nausea, and light sensitivity that can impair your life. When traditional treatments fall short, many patients seek alternative therapies like acupuncture and acupressure to find comfort. In this research, we will dig into the intriguing realm of these ancient therapeutic traditions and learn how they provide a beacon of hope for migraine patients.

HOW ACUPUNCTURE WORKS FOR MIGRAINES:

Imagine microscopic, hair-thin needles softly implanted into particular locations on your body. This may seem like the opening scene of a horror movie, but it's really the essence of acupuncture, an ancient Chinese therapeutic method that has been utilized for millennia. Acupuncture tries to balance the flow of vital energy, or "qi" (pronounced "chee"), via meridians in the body. When it comes to migraines, this strategy may be a game-changer.

Qi Flow and Migraines:
In traditional Chinese medicine, migraines are commonly related to interruptions in the flow of qi. Acupuncture tries to restore equilibrium by placing needles into exact places along the meridians linked with migraine relief. These locations activate the neurological system, causing the release of natural analgesics like endorphins and serotonin. They also soothe stiff muscles and increase blood circulation.

Holistic Healing:
What makes acupuncture so intriguing is its comprehensive approach. It doesn't simply

target the symptoms but treats the fundamental causes of migraines. This means an acupuncturist could inquire about your nutrition, stress levels, and sleep habits to develop a treatment plan that meets your individual requirements.

Frequency and Consistency:
While some individuals feel instant alleviation, others may need repeated sessions for enduring effects. Regular acupuncture treatments might not only lessen the frequency and severity of migraines but also boost your general well-being.

PRESSURE POINTS FOR MIGRAINE RELIEF:
If needles make you squirm, don't fear — acupressure is a fantastic option. It includes employing hard pressure with your fingers or thumbs on targeted locations rather than

needles. Here are some helpful pressure locations for migraine relief:

Taiyang (Extra 1):
Located near the temples, the Taiyang point is an effective site for reducing migraine discomfort. Gently massage this region in a circular manner to relax stiff muscles and stimulate blood flow.

Hegu (LI4):
Found between the thumb and index finger, Hegu is known as the "Great Eliminator." Applying strong pressure here may help lower headache severity and potentially avoid migraines.

Yintang (Extra 2):
Positioned between the eyebrows, Yintang is commonly termed the "Third Eye Point." Applying continuous pressure to this point helps ease tension and stress that lead to headaches.

Fengchi (GB20):
These points are placed near the base of your head, on each side of your spine. Massaging them helps lessen neck strain and improve migraine symptoms.

Zusanli (ST36):
Situated on the lower thigh, Zusanli may aid with general headache treatment by inducing relaxation and boosting circulation.

In conclusion, acupuncture and acupressure provide intriguing options for migraine patients seeking natural, drug-free therapies. These traditional healing methods concentrate on harmonizing your body's energy flow and treating the underlying causes of migraines. Whether you select acupuncture's precision needling or acupressure's gentle pressure, these treatments provide a glimmer of hope for people seeking relief from the pounding anguish of migraines.

CHIROPRACTIC CARE
- Alignment and Nervous System
- Chiropractic Approaches for Migraine Relief

what if I told you that relief may be found in a place you would not anticipate — your local chiropractor's office? Chiropractic therapy, traditionally linked with spine adjustments, has a hidden gem of possible migraine relief. In this investigation, we'll look into how chiropractic therapy affects the alignment of your spine and neurological system to reduce migraines. So, gear yourself for a fascinating voyage into the realm of chiropractic techniques for migraine relief.

ALIGNMENT AND NERVOUS SYSTEM FOR MIGRAINE RELIEF:
To understand how chiropractic therapy might help reduce migraines, let's start with the spine — a flexible yet robust column of bones that contains the delicate network of

nerves known as the nervous system. This system, encompassing the brain, spinal cord, and many nerves branching throughout your body, plays a key role in your general well-being, including migraine management.

Misalignments And Migraines: Chiropractors think that misalignments or subluxations in the spine might inhibit the appropriate passage of information along the nervous system.
These misalignments may come from different things including poor posture, stress, injury, or simply the wear and tear of regular living. When these subluxations occur at the upper cervical spine (the neck), they might possibly induce or intensify migraine symptoms.

Restoring Balance: Chiropractors employ particular methods to gently manipulate and adjust the spine, seeking to rectify these subluxations. This not only assists in restoring normal spinal alignment but also encourages improved communication throughout the neurological system. When the neurological system performs correctly, it might possibly lessen the frequency and severity of migraine attacks.

CHIROPRACTIC APPROACHES FOR MIGRAINE RELIEF:
Now that we understand the role of spinal alignment and the neurological system in migraine treatment, let's dig into the chiropractic techniques that might help:

- Spinal Adjustments: This is the hallmark of chiropractic therapy. By utilizing controlled, manual force, chiropractors realign the vertebrae of the spine. When aimed at particular locations connected to migraine triggers, such as the neck and upper back, these adjustments may give great relief.

- Posture and Lifestyle Counseling: Chiropractors don't stop at spinal adjustments. They typically teach patients about keeping appropriate postures and implementing healthy lifestyle behaviors. Simple improvements like ergonomically constructed workstations and exercises to strengthen neck and back muscles may help prevent the frequency of migraines.
- Dietary Guidance: Some chiropractors also give dietary counseling. Certain foods or dietary habits may function as migraine triggers for certain persons. By adopting suitable dietary modifications, people may suffer fewer migraines.
- Stress Management: Stress is a typical migraine cause. Chiropractors commonly include stress-reduction treatments such as relaxation exercises or mindfulness practices in their treatment programs.

- **Holistic Approach:** Many chiropractors use a holistic approach, addressing the complete body's health and well-being. This holistic approach may include conversations about sleep habits, hydration, and other variables that potentially impact migraine incidence.

In conclusion, chiropractic therapy for migraines provides a comprehensive, non-invasive way to manage this terrible illness. By concentrating on spinal alignment and nervous system function, chiropractors strive to minimize the frequency and severity of migraine episodes.

While not a one-size-fits-all treatment, many migraine patients have found considerable relief and increased quality of life with chiropractic therapy. So, if migraines have been keeping you captive, try exploring the realm of chiropractic treatment — it could just be the key to unlocking a migraine-free future.

AROMATHERAPY AND ESSENTIAL OILS
- Essential Oils for Migraine Relief
- Aromatherapy Techniques

While pharmaceuticals are frequently the first line of defense, there's a relaxing, natural option worth trying — aromatherapy and essential oils. Imagine finding respite from the persistent grip of a migraine via the power of smells and oils.

In this voyage into the realm of aromatherapy, we'll expose the mysteries of essential oils for migraine treatment and explore the efficient aromatherapy practices that may help ease your pain, all while making the process both engaging and simple to grasp.

ESSENTIAL OILS FOR MIGRAINE RELIEF:

- Lavender Oil: Often called the crown gem of essential oils, lavender oil contains exceptional relaxing effects. Its relaxing scent might help reduce the stress that sometimes accompanies migraines. Simply inhaling lavender oil or mixing it with a carrier oil and putting it to your temples may bring comfort.
- Peppermint Oil: Peppermint oil is a formidable ally in the battle against migraines. Its cooling effect and analgesic characteristics may help lower headache severity. Applying diluted peppermint oil to your forehead or breathing it deeply might work miracles.
- Rosemary Oil: Known for its capacity to enhance blood circulation, rosemary oil might be your go-to oil for fighting migraine-related symptoms. Gently massage diluted

rosemary oil over your neck and shoulders to relax tight muscles and minimize headache symptoms.

- Eucalyptus Oil: Eucalyptus oil's stimulating aroma may help remove congestion and promote oxygen flow, making it an excellent alternative for migraine treatment, particularly when congestion exacerbates your migraines. Diffuse it or inhale its vapor to feel its advantages.

- Chamomile Oil: Chamomile oil's anti-inflammatory and relaxation-inducing qualities may help reduce migraines. You may sip on chamomile tea or use chamomile oil in a steam inhalation to reduce stress and pain.

AROMATHERAPY TECHNIQUES FOR MIGRAINES:

- Diffusion: Aromatherapy diffusers are a popular approach to disseminating essential oils into the air. Choose an essential oil or combination that meets your tastes and let the diffuser perform its magic. As you breathe in the scented mist, you'll find relief from your migraine symptoms.

- Topical Application: Dilute your selected essential oil with a carrier oil, such as jojoba or coconut oil, and apply it to your pulse points or the regions where you feel stress, such as your temples, neck, and shoulders. The oil will be absorbed via your skin, delivering both a relaxing aroma and physical comfort.
- Steam Inhalation: Boil a kettle of water, add a few drops of your choice essential oil, and gently inhale the steam with a towel wrapped over your head. This approach may help free up your nasal passages and relieve congestion, offering relief from migraine-related sinus pain.
- Aromatic Baths: Add a few drops of your selected essential oil to a warm

bath and immerse yourself in the calming smell. This procedure not only relaxes your body but also enables the oil to infiltrate your skin, boosting relaxation and reducing headache symptoms.

- Personal Inhalers: Portable inhalers filled with essential oils are available for on-the-go treatment. Simply breathe via the gadget anytime a migraine begins to attack.

In the realm of migraines, where pain and suffering typically take center stage, aromatherapy and essential oils provide a comprehensive approach to healing. These natural medicines give not only physical relief but also mental tranquillity, making your migraine trip a little more tolerable.

With a range of essential oils and aromatherapy methods at your disposal, you may begin on a fragrant journey towards a brighter, headache-free future. So, take a deep breath, let the fragrances transport you away, and allow aromatherapy and essential oils to be your friends in the struggle against migraines.

TRADITIONAL CHINESE MEDICINE (TCM) APPROACHES
- Herbal Formulas in TCM
- Acupuncture in TCM

Traditional Chinese Medicine (TCM) provides a novel and holistic method of managing migraines. At the core of TCM lies a rich mine of ancient knowledge that mixes herbal formulae with acupuncture, providing not only healing but a better understanding of the body's subtle balance.

HERBAL FORMULAS IN TCM FOR MIGRAINES

Imagine a world where nature holds the answer to your migraine treatment. In TCM, this idea is far from a fantasy; it's a well-practiced reality. Herbal formulae, commonly recommended as teas or powders, are important to TCM's approach to migraine therapy. The answer lies in treating the fundamental causes of the headaches, not merely hiding the discomfort.

Chuan Xiong Cha Tiao San: Picture this herbal treatment as a calm wind that clears away the clouds of headache. Chuan Xiong Cha Tiao San, combining Chuan Xiong (Szechuan lovage root) and Bo He (mint), works wonderfully for migraines induced by stagnated Qi and blood circulation. It relaxes the arteries and unblocks the channels that contribute to those throbbing aches.

Ling Jiao Gou Teng Tang: If your migraines seem like a raging tempest within your mind, Ling Jiao Gou Teng Tang might be your lifeline. Made from the potent combination of Gou Teng (Uncaria stem) and Ling Yang Jiao (antelope horn), this compound calms the liver and extinguishes the fire that could be causing your migraines. It's like a refreshing shower on a sweltering summer day.

Xiao Yao San: Sometimes, migraines develop from stress and mental distress, and that's where Xiao Yao San comes in. Comprising herbs like Bai Shao (white peony) and Chai Hu (bupleurum), it harmonizes the mind and body, helping you to find serenity despite the storm.

But how can you know which formula is suitable for you? That's where TCM's individualized approach shines. A professional TCM practitioner will examine your particular constitution, the type of your migraines, and any underlying imbalances before prescribing the correct herbal mix for you.

ACUPUNCTURE IN TCM FOR MIGRAINES

Now, picture a world where small needles may disperse the clouds of migraine torment. That's the miracle of acupuncture, a cornerstone of TCM. Acupuncture sees migraines as interruptions in the flow of Qi, or vital energy, through the body's meridians. By precisely placing ultra-fine needles at certain acupoints, TCM practitioners try to reestablish this flow and deliver comfort.

Taiyang and Fengchi sites: These sites, positioned at the base of the skull and the temple respectively, are like pressure valves for migraine treatment. Stimulating them may ease the acute pain and pressure that typically accompanies migraines.

Neiguan Point: Nestled in the crease of your wrist, the Neiguan Point may perform wonders for tension headaches. Activating this acupoint helps calm the body and reduce stress-related migraines.

Hegu Point: Found between the thumb and index finger, this acupoint is a potent ally against migraines. It's thought to ease pain and lessen stress throughout the body.

But acupuncture is more than just a simple placement of needles; it's a precise technique. TCM practitioners meticulously customize each session to your unique symptoms, ensuring that the energy balance in your body is restored, making it less prone to future migraine episodes.

In the realm of TCM, migraines are not simply headaches to be numbed; they're messages from your body, screaming for balance and harmony.

By digging into the age-old understanding of herbal formulations and acupuncture, TCM opens the doors to a comprehensive approach that not only alleviates migraines but supports your whole well-being. So, next time a migraine cloud approaches your sky, remember that Traditional Chinese Medicine provides a road to tranquility despite the storm.

CHAPTER 4

<u>MIGRAINES & DIET: What You Should Know</u>

EXPLORING THE LINK BETWEEN DIET AND MIGRAINES

In the area of medical study, the relationship between nutrition and migraines has emerged as an intriguing and ever-evolving issue. Migraines are not simply typical headaches; they are complicated neurological processes that impact millions of individuals worldwide. For decades, experts have been fascinated by the concept that our food choices can play a major role in the onset, frequency, and severity of these debilitating episodes.

So, let's begin on a voyage into the exciting realm of migraines and food. We'll investigate the science underlying this link, find frequent dietary triggers, and discover the items that could bring help. As we go further, you'll discover that the relationship between nutrition and migraines is not simply a question of what's on your plate; it's a window into knowing your own body, its sensitivities, and the ability you possess to possibly regulate these terrible episodes. Let's plunge in and make sense of this interesting puzzle, piece by piece.

The Brain's Cry For Help
Before we go into the enticing relationship between what we eat and headaches, let's take a minute to grasp what a migraine truly is. A migraine is not simply a headache; it's a neurovascular illness marked by strong, throbbing pain, typically accompanied by additional unpleasant symptoms such as nausea, vomiting, and sensitivity to light and sound.

While the specific etiology of migraines remains a matter of continuing study, they are thought to involve the brain and blood vessels. When a migraine episode develops, there is a complicated interaction of chemical signals, inflammation, and changes in blood flow inside the brain. Think of it as the brain's scream for aid, suggesting that something is awry.

But what does this have to do with your diet? Well, the foods and drinks you eat may have a tremendous influence on the brain's chemistry and blood flow, thereby impacting the onset and intensity of migraine episodes. This is when the fascinating relationship between nutrition and migraines starts to take form.

Food: Friend or Foe?
Our diets are a key component of our life. They bring food, enjoyment, and occasionally, even a feeling of comfort. But what if the foods we enjoy might also be the perpetrators behind those excruciating migraines? It's a surprising idea and one

that researchers have been painstakingly examining.

Certain meals and drinks have emerged as suspected migraine causes. These dietary villains might differ from person to person, making the relationship between food and migraines all the more interesting and individualized. For some, it may be a glass of red wine; for others, it might be that treasured piece of chocolate cake. Understanding your particular food triggers may be like solving a jigsaw, and it may contain the key to avoiding future migraines.

However, not all hope is gone. Just as some foods could induce migraines, others might act as your friends in the fight against these severe headaches. The notion of "diet therapy" for migraines is gaining popularity as experts uncover that certain meals offer the capacity to calm and prevent these episodes.

Unraveling the Mystery

The relationship between nutrition and migraines is a complicated puzzle, waiting to be uncovered. In this inquiry, we will trek through the maze of scientific data, separating myth from fact, and obtaining insights into how what you eat might affect your migraine experience.

As we journey through the realm of dietary triggers and possible cures, you'll learn practical techniques and tactics to control your migraines via food choices. Whether you're a migraine sufferer seeking treatment or just inquisitive about the delicate link between nutrition and health, this trip promises to capture your curiosity and empower you with information.

So, strap your seatbelts, because we are about to go on a fascinating adventure into the domain of nutrition and migraines, where each meal is a piece of the jigsaw and every mouthful contains the potential to reveal the secrets of treating and, maybe, even overcoming this puzzling neurological illness.

TRIGGER FOODS: UNLOCKING THE MYSTERY OF MIGRAINE CULPRITS

While migraines might have different causes, one surprise culprit frequently lies in plain sight: your diet. Yes, you heard it correctly! Common meals and components may be subtle migraine instigators, turning your enjoyable dinner into a terrible nightmare. In this tour into the labyrinth of migraine-triggering foods, we'll explore the secrets behind the likes of MSG, caffeine, and artificial sweeteners.

MSG (Monosodium Glutamate): The Umami Bombshell

MSG, the renowned flavor enhancer present in many commercial and restaurant meals, could possibly be the sneakiest migraine cause of all. Often included under the disguise of "natural flavors" or "hydrolyzed protein" on ingredient labels, MSG may drive your mind into a dizzying spiral. How does it work? MSG overstimulates nerve cells, resulting in increased brain activity - the ideal prescription for a migraine. So, next time you're eating that delectable bowl of quick noodles or a savory restaurant meal, be careful of the hidden umami bombshell lying inside.

Caffeine: The Double-Edged Sword
For many, caffeine is the morning elixir, bringing a much-needed energy boost. But for migraine patients, it's a double-edged sword. While a modest dosage of coffee might occasionally help headaches, too much can throw you into a migraine loop. The key is balance.
Overindulgence may lead to withdrawal headaches, whereas sudden caffeine withdrawal can be an even more important cause. So, whether it's your morning coffee or an afternoon pick-me-up, keep caffeine

consumption in control to stay ahead of those migraines.

Artificial Sweeteners: The Sweet, Silent Saboteurs

Artificial sweeteners like aspartame and sucralose look like a gift for dieters, giving sweetness without calories.

However, they have a bad side when it comes to migraines. These sugar replacements may disturb brain chemistry, changing serotonin levels and laying the scene for a migraine reprise. So, diet Coke or sugar-free gum can be guilty pleasures that come with a severe price. Opting for natural sweeteners like stevia or just limiting your sweet desire may be a safer choice.

Tyramine: The Fermented Foe

Tyramine is a naturally occurring chemical found in aged and fermented foods including cheese, red wine, and soy sauce. While these delights please the palette, they may wreak havoc for migraine-prone people. Tyramine promotes the release of norepinephrine, a neurotransmitter related to headaches. So, if you're planning a romantic supper with wine and cheese, consider the possible ramifications for your brain before indulging too heavily.

Nitrites and Nitrates: The Deli Dilemma
Those delectable deli meats and bacon you love so much may also be adding to your migraine pain. They commonly include nitrites and nitrates, preservatives needed to keep color and taste. Unfortunately, these substances may widen blood vessels and contribute to migraines. Consider selecting nitrate-free options to shield yourself from this deli issue.

Understanding which meals and components might be your migraine adversary is a voyage of self-discovery. Keeping a food journal may be tremendously useful in recognizing your individual triggers. By recognizing and eliminating these common offenders like MSG, caffeine, artificial sweeteners, tyramine, nitrites, and nitrates, and being diligent about food additives and preservatives, you may take control of your migraines and restore a life free from the shackles of terrible headaches.

In this examination of trigger foods, we've exposed the various factors behind migraines, providing light on how apparently benign components may transform a dinner into a migraine agony. Remember, information is power, and recognizing these triggers may be your weapon against the tyranny of migraines. So, as you continue on your path to overcoming these terrible episodes, may you navigate the culinary world with intelligence and live a life filled with fewer migraine storms.

WHAT IS A FOOD DIARY AND HOW CAN YOU USE IT?

Migraines are complicated and mysterious. Their origins differ from person to person, making it tough to establish the specific reason. For some, it's stress; for others, it's hormone swings. But what if your migraines were silently hidden in the food you eat daily?

This is when the beauty of food diaries comes into play. A food diary is more than simply a record of what you eat; it's a thorough notebook that captures everything from the minute food touches your lips to the commencement of a migraine episode. But why is it so important?

The Importance of Keeping a Food Diary
Personalization: No two migraines are identical, and the causes might be as unique as your fingerprints. What brings off a migraine for you may not affect someone else. A food diary helps you tailor your migraine therapy by determining the exact

meals or substances that function as your own migraine triggers.

Pattern Recognition: Migraines generally follow patterns, and these patterns might be discovered by thorough record-keeping. By monitoring your food consumption, you might uncover patterns, such as certain foods or combinations that typically precede a migraine episode.

Empowerment: Knowledge is power. Armed with the information from your food journal, you have the upper hand in controlling your migraines. You may make educated decisions about what to eat and what to avoid, minimizing the frequency and severity of your episodes.

Communication with Healthcare Providers: When you see a healthcare practitioner about your migraines, maintaining a thorough food diary may be a game-changer. It delivers actual proof of your triggers, permitting a more precise diagnosis and treatment strategy.

Holistic Health: Your dietary choices affect not just your migraines but also your entire health. By maintaining a food diary, you become more observant of your eating choices, perhaps leading to a better lifestyle.

Starting Your Food Diary Journey
Creating a food journal is quite straightforward. All you need is a notepad or a digital app to capture the following information:

- Date and hour of each meal or snack.
- Detailed descriptions of everything you eat and drink, including portion quantities.
- Any symptoms or migraine episodes, including their strength and length.

As you consistently keep your food diary, you'll begin to observe connections between your diet and your migraines. These links may not be immediately visible, but with time, patterns will develop, giving you crucial insights into your particular migraine triggers.

Remember, finding your particular migraine triggers with a food diary is a process that demands time and effort. It's a voyage of self-discovery that may lead to a happier, migraine-free future. So, grab that pen download that app, and begin on this powerful adventure to unearth the mysteries concealed on your plate. Your migraine-free existence may be only a few diary entries away!

NAVIGATING THE SUGAR-MIGRAINE CONNECTION

Imagine this scenario: you're experiencing a sweet tooth need, and that piece of cake or chocolate bar is screaming your name. You indulge yourself, relishing the sweet bliss, but suddenly, out of nowhere, a migraine hits. That pounding headache, nausea, and sensitivity to light and sound may spoil your day. Is there a relationship between sugar and migraines? Let's dig into the sweet science of this often-overlooked link and uncover how sugar intake can impact the frequency and intensity of those annoying migraines.

Sugar Rush and the Brain:
First, let's grasp how sugar impacts our bodies, particularly our brains. When you ingest sugar, your blood sugar levels jump. This fast influx of glucose in your system delivers a short burst of energy. However, your body doesn't enjoy this sugar rollercoaster trip. To combat the elevated sugar levels, it produces insulin, a hormone that helps control blood sugar. As a consequence, your blood sugar drops, typically leading to feelings of exhaustion and anger.

Now, consider your brain in this sugar drama. It's a sensitive organ that depends largely on a regular supply of glucose for energy. When blood sugar levels change quickly, your brain might become agitated, and this stress can possibly produce headaches in certain people. Studies have revealed that these variations might possibly contribute to abnormalities in blood flow, inflammation, and even chemical imbalances in the brain, all of which are connected to migraine development.

Sugar and Inflammation:
Inflammation is a buzzword in the world of health and with good reason. Chronic inflammation has been related to several health concerns, including migraines. Sugar, notably the refined variety found in sweets and processed meals, is a proven pro-inflammatory agent. It may lead to higher levels of inflammation throughout your body, particularly in the blood vessels and brain.

For migraine patients, this inflammatory reaction might be a trigger. Inflammation may irritate nerves, resulting in the pounding pain that defines migraines. Moreover, it may make the brain more sensitive to pain, perhaps worsening the intensity of your headache.

Sugar & Hormonal Rollercoasters:
Hormones have a key influence on migraines, especially in women. Fluctuations in estrogen levels are typically connected with migraine headaches. Interestingly, sugar may impact these hormonal rollercoasters.

When you eat significant quantities of sugar, it may lead to insulin resistance, which can, in turn, impact hormone levels, particularly in women. This hormonal imbalance may contribute to the frequency and severity of migraines.

The Sugar-Migraine Connection:

While the association between sugar and migraines isn't crystal clear, there is accumulating evidence to show that sugar intake may definitely increase the frequency and severity of migraine episodes. It's vital to understand that migraines are complicated, and numerous events might cause them. Sugar is simply one element of the puzzle.

So, if you're prone to migraines, it could be worth evaluating your sugar consumption. Reducing your intake of sugary snacks and opting for a balanced diet might perhaps help decrease the frequency and severity of those awful headaches. However, it's vital to speak with a healthcare practitioner for specialized guidance on controlling your migraines.

In conclusion, the sweet delight of sugar may bring brief pleasure, but it might also be harboring a dark secret - a possible relationship to the terrible migraine. While research continues to unearth the nuances of this link, being careful of your sugar consumption and its implications on your general health is a sensible option. So, next time you grab for that sugary pleasure, you may want to consider the message your body, and your brain, are telling you — a sweet treat now can imply a pounding headache tomorrow.

CAFFEINE AND MIGRAINES: EXPLORING THE INTRICATE CONNECTION

Ah, caffeine – that lovely pick-me-up found in our morning coffee, beloved sodas, and even chocolate. For many of us, it's the reliable partner to our daily routine, delivering a surge of energy when we need it most. But for individuals who fight with the searing, head-splitting misery of migraines, coffee isn't always the hero it appears to be. In reality, it could simply be a double-edged sword.

In this research, we're delving deep into the interesting association between coffee and migraines. It's a narrative of highs and lows, a tale of reliance and withdrawal, and a desire for balance among the turmoil. Migraines, those dreadful headaches that may leave even the mightiest among us gripping our temples in despair, have been the focus of innumerable research. But coffee, that sneaky stimulant hiding in our regular drinks, remains an elusive figure in the migraine tale.

So, what's the thing with coffee and migraines? How does coffee consumption affect these pulsing nightmares that strike some of us much too frequently? What happens when we attempt to stop caffeine? And most crucially, can we develop a method to cohabit with coffee without inducing migraines? Grab your favorite caffeinated beverage, sit back, and join us on this exciting trip through the caffeine-migraine link. We're going to solve the enigma, drink by sip.

For many migraine patients, coffee might feel like a savior. When a migraine comes in, a cup of coffee or a caffeine-containing pain treatment could bring fast relief. Caffeine constricts blood vessels and decreases inflammation, which may help lessen the pounding anguish that defines migraines. It may boost the efficacy of certain over-the-counter pain drugs too.

However, as they say, "Too much of a good thing can be bad," and this couldn't be truer when it comes to coffee and migraines. Regular, excessive coffee consumption might really become a migraine cause. It's a bizarre position where what formerly gave solace might now be the originator of your suffering.

Caffeine Intake and Migraine Onset

So, how can coffee, which gives reprieve during a migraine episode, transform into a migraine culprit? It all comes down to the body's delicate equilibrium and the phenomena of withdrawal.

When you ingest caffeine consistently, your body develops acclimated to its presence. Over time, you may find yourself requiring more coffee to have the same invigorating impact. This is the famed caffeine tolerance. However, when you abruptly cut or cease your caffeine consumption, the pendulum swings the opposite way - you suffer caffeine withdrawal.

Caffeine withdrawal is the body's method of reacting against the absent stimulant. As the caffeine levels decrease, your blood vessels widen, leading to greater blood flow to the brain. This abrupt shift in vascular tone may produce a migraine episode, commonly accompanied by unmistakable throbbing pain, sensitivity to light and sound, and nausea.

The Withdrawal Headache
The withdrawal headache, which may resemble a full-blown migraine, is a common indication of caffeine withdrawal. It normally kicks in between 12 to 24 hours of lowering or discontinuing coffee. The intensity may vary from slight discomfort to a head-splitting experience, depending on your coffee use patterns and individual sensitivity.

What's particularly remarkable is that if you're a habitual caffeine user and you try to cut down, you may not even identify your current headaches with caffeine withdrawal. It's a brilliant deception perpetrated by your brain, seeking to cajole you into renewing its coffee fix.

Navigating the Caffeine-Migraine Maze

So, where does this leave us in the caffeine-migraine conundrum? Is caffeine a friend or adversary for migraine sufferers? Well, it's both. In moderation, coffee could give relief during a migraine episode. However, it's crucial to be cautious of your caffeine consumption and not let it become a crutch. If you find yourself in a vicious cycle of caffeine dependency and withdrawal headaches, it may be time to gradually lower your caffeine consumption.

Migraines are complicated, and their triggers may differ from person to person. For some, coffee may really be a powerful trigger, while for others, it may bring occasional reprieve. Understanding your body's particular interaction with coffee is a vital step in controlling migraine episodes efficiently.

In this path of coffee and migraines, moderation and awareness are your friends. As you drink your coffee or go for that chocolate bar, remember that caffeine is like a perfectly tuned instrument, capable of playing both soothing and dissonant notes in the symphony of your life. Balancing the act is the key to ensuring that caffeine stays a friend and not an adversary in your struggle against migraines.

THE GLUTEN & MIGRAINE ENIGMA: is there a relationship

What is Gluten?

Gluten is a protein compound found in cereals including wheat, barley, and rye. It's the glue that keeps your dough together, making it supple and elastic. This adaptable protein may be found in numerous culinary products, from bread and pasta to sauces, soups, and even some surprising locations like cosmetics and pharmaceuticals.

What are Migraines?

Migraines are not your garden-variety headaches. They're more like thunderstorms within your head. These neurological storms may bring pounding pain, nausea, vomiting, and sensitivity to light and sound. For individuals who suffer from migraines, they may be totally debilitating, making even the simplest chores appear Herculean.

Now, let's cut to the chase: what's the relationship between gluten and these awful migraines?

The Gluten Sensitivity Puzzle
For some folks, ingesting gluten isn't all sunshine and rainbows. They could suffer a spectrum of symptoms commonly called "gluten sensitivity." These symptoms can vary greatly, from digestive troubles to weariness and, yeah, you got it, headaches.

While gluten sensitivity isn't as severe as celiac disease (an autoimmune ailment induced by gluten), it's still a likely reason for those inexplicable migraine headaches. Some experts think that gluten sensitivity might contribute to persistent inflammation in the body, harming blood vessels and neurons, which are crucial players in the migraine game.

The Celiac Disease Connection
Now, let's zero in on celiac disease—a significantly more dangerous ailment. When someone with celiac disease eats gluten, their immune system goes wild, attacking the lining of the small intestine. But here's the twist in our migraine tale: celiac disease doesn't simply end at the stomach. It may unleash pandemonium throughout the body, including the brain.

Celiac disease commonly goes hand in hand with neurological symptoms, with migraines being one of them. The particular processes aren't entirely known, but it's thought that the immune system's reaction to gluten might produce these excruciating headaches.

Unmasking the Migraine-Gluten Link

So, what's the judgment on the probable relationship between gluten sensitivity, celiac disease, and migraines? Well, it's still a bit of a scientific riddle. While some persons with gluten sensitivity or celiac disease report a considerable decrease in migraines when they follow a gluten-free diet, not everyone experiences this miraculous cure.

What we do know is that for a subgroup of migraine patients, gluten could be a hidden antagonist. The link is complicated and extremely personalized, making it vital to contact a healthcare physician if you suspect a gluten-migraine connection in your life. They can assist you in negotiating dietary modifications and uncover possible triggers to control those migraine storms.

In conclusion, the gluten-migraine riddle continues to excite experts and migraine patients alike. While it may not contain all the solutions to the conundrum of migraines, it's an interesting piece of the jigsaw that underlines the delicate interaction between nutrition, the immune system, and the brain. So, the next time you grab that slice of pizza and your head begins pounding, ponder the gluten-migraine connection—a little but interesting piece of the greater migraine enigma.

THE ANTI-INFLAMMATORY DIET: YOUR SHIELD AGAINST MIGRAINE ATTACKS

Inflammation is the body's normal reaction to injury or sickness, but when it becomes chronic and systemic, it may wreak havoc on our health. Think of it as a fire that never fully burns out, simmering under the surface and wreaking damage over time. And here's where the anti-inflammatory diet comes in, equipped with an assortment of foods that may help extinguish that chronic fire, perhaps leading to fewer migraine days and a dramatically enhanced quality of life.

So, how does it work? By concentrating on foods that lower inflammation, you're effectively taking away the fuel that feeds the migraine beast. Inflammatory foods, on the other hand, operate as a firestarter, starting those painful episodes with every meal. It's a gastronomic tug-of-war between what you select to put on your plate and how your body reacts.

But what are these mythical anti-inflammatory foods, and which villains should you shun from your diet? Think of it this way: you're seeking to build a cuisine that's high in antioxidants, omega-3 fatty acids, and a rainbow of fruits and vegetables. These superheroes of the culinary world work diligently to neutralize those inflammatory substances, calming the inflamed nerves that might lead to migraine mayhem.

On the other side, inflammatory foods include the typical suspects: sugary delights, processed snacks, and an oversupply of red meat. These dietary delinquents are known to stir the embers of inflammation, possibly kindling the next migraine episode.

Now, it's crucial to remember that although an anti-inflammatory diet may not be a definite migraine cure, it may undoubtedly be a strong ally in your struggle against these terrible headaches. By adopting this culinary strategy, you're equipping yourself with a natural defense, one that may drastically lessen the frequency and severity of migraines, and possibly even offer the hope of a life free from the tyranny of continual head pain.

Now, let's speak about the hero of our narrative - the anti-inflammatory diet. This isn't simply another fad diet; it's a lifestyle shift that is centered on ingesting foods that may help decrease inflammation in the body. By doing so, it becomes your secret weapon against migraines. How does it work, you ask?

Bye-Bye Inflammatory Foods
Imagine your body as a war. In one corner, you have inflammatory foods like processed snacks, sugary delights, and trans fats - the villains that cause inflammation. In the opposite corner, you have the heroes of the anti-inflammatory diet: fresh fruits, vegetables, whole grains, fatty fish, and nuts. When you cut those inflammatory items out of your diet and replace them with their anti-inflammatory equivalents, you're effectively disarming the adversary and reinforcing your defenses.

Omega-3 Fatty Acids:
Fatty seafood like salmon, mackerel, and sardines are your friends in your combat against migraines. They're filled with omega-3 fatty acids, which are effective anti-inflammatories. These good fats assist in regulating blood flow, decrease

inflammation in blood vessels, and may even diminish the frequency and severity of migraine episodes.

Antioxidant Avengers:
Fruits and vegetables are filled with antioxidants like vitamins C and E, which neutralize damaging free radicals and reduce inflammation. Berries, in particular, are like small, delectable warriors in this struggle. Their abundant antioxidants may give protection against migraine triggers.

The Spice of Life
Turmeric, with its main component curcumin, is a spice noted for its outstanding anti-inflammatory qualities. Incorporating turmeric into your meals might be a game-changer for migraine prevention. It's like having a superhero shielding your head from the approaching storm.

The Hydration Hero:

Don't underestimate the power of water. Dehydration may lead to inflammation, and inflammation can provoke migraines. Staying well-hydrated is a simple but efficient strategy to keep migraines at bay.

So, if you've ever fantasized about a world without migraines, where your mind is clear and free from anguish, try making the anti-inflammatory diet your loyal friend. It's not simply a method of eating; it's a lifestyle shift that may lead to a future filled with fewer gloomy rooms, less pain, and more pleasure. So, why not start on this gastronomic journey and learn how the power of food may help you beat the migraine monster, one mouthful at a time? Your mind, and your life, could just thank you for it.

THE CULPRITS: FOOD ALLERGIES VS. FOOD SENSITIVITIES

Before we enter into the migraine-mystery-solving adventure, let's differentiate between two essential players: food allergies and food sensitivities.

Food Allergies: These are like the detectives of the food world, with your immune system as the smart investigator. When you ingest anything you're allergic to (such as peanuts or shellfish), your immune system goes on high alert, treating the allergen as a harmful invader.

It releases a multitude of chemicals, including histamines, which may cause quick, severe symptoms like hives, swelling, or trouble breathing. Food allergies are often identified by skin testing, blood tests, or oral food challenges.

Food Sensitivities: Think of food sensitivities as the sneakier perpetrators. Unlike allergies, sensitivities don't provoke an instant immunological reaction. Instead, they lead to delayed and generally milder effects. These may include digestion troubles, skin problems, and yep, you got it, migraines. Identifying food sensitivities may be hard since there's no one-size-fits-all test. It generally includes an elimination diet, when you eliminate particular items from your diet and reintroduce them one at a time to observe how your body responds.

Unmasking the Migraine Triggers: Food and Migraines
Now, let's get to the core of the matter: how can food allergies and sensitivities create those annoying migraines?

Inflammatory Response: Both food allergies and sensitivities may contribute to inflammation in the body. When this inflammation develops in the blood vessels and nerves surrounding your brain, it might create the foundation for a migraine attack. Certain meals, including processed meats and sugary snacks, are renowned for increasing inflammation.

Histamine Havoc: Histamines, produced during allergic responses, may also be headache reasons. Foods strong in histamine, such as aged cheeses, smoked meats, and fermented drinks, might induce migraines in persons sensitive to this chemical.

Vasoactive Amines: Some foods include vasoactive amines like tyramine, which may cause blood vessels to tighten and then quickly dilate. This blood vessel rollercoaster might cause migraine headaches. Foods like old cheeses, red wine, and certain processed meats are high in tyramine.

Trigger Variability: It's crucial to realize that migraine triggers may vary greatly from person to person. What causes one individual a throbbing headache could not affect another at all. This heterogeneity might make identifying dietary triggers problematic, but it also underscores the necessity of tailored approaches to migraine therapy.

Detective Work: Identifying Your Food Migraine Triggers

Now that we've established the science behind it, let's explore how to play detective and determine your unique dietary migraine triggers:

Keep a Food Diary: Document what you eat and when you have migraines. Patterns may develop, letting you discover likely offenders.

Elimination Diet: Under the advice of a healthcare expert or a certified dietitian, go on an elimination diet. Gradually reintroduce foods one by one to check whether they provoke migraines.

Consider Testing: While not definite, certain testing like IgG food sensitivity tests might give insights into probable causes. However, these tests have limitations and should be interpreted carefully.

Migraine-Free Living: Managing Food Allergies and Sensitivities

Once you've solved the case and discovered your dietary triggers, it's time to enjoy a migraine-free life:

Adapt Your Diet: Remove or minimize the migraine-triggering items from your diet. Focus on complete, unprocessed meals, and remain hydrated.

Stay Consistent: Migraine treatment is a lengthy game. Stay persistent with your dietary adjustments, since it might take time to observe gains.

Lifestyle Factors: Don't forget about other migraine factors including stress, lack of sleep, and dehydration. Addressing these issues might complement your dietary modifications.

In conclusion, food allergies and sensitivities are like secret saboteurs in the realm of migraines. By recognizing their function and beginning on a detective quest to find your specific triggers, you may take control of your migraines and move towards a life free from terrible headaches. Remember, it's a journey, but the destination—a migraine-free life—is worth every step.

MIGRAINE-FRIENDLY RECIPES FOR YOU

Migraine patients know all too well that some foods may function as silent instigators of their suffering. These triggers, ranging from chemical additives to particular kinds of cheese or alcohol, may wreak havoc on delicate neurovascular systems. However, there's no need to lose taste and pleasure on your quest towards fewer migraines. With this comprehensive recipe collection, we've carefully picked foods that not only tickle your taste senses but also respect your well-being.

In the pages that follow, you'll find a plethora of dishes that cater to the special dietary demands of migraineurs. We've adopted a holistic approach that reduces possible migraine triggers while optimizing flavor and nutritional value. From breakfast to dessert, our dishes are meant to make your gastronomic journey as pleasurable as possible, without the fear of looming headaches.

Our attitude is simple: "No more migraines, but more flavor." You'll discover recipes that switch out troublesome components with migraine-friendly alternatives, guaranteeing you may enjoy your favorite foods with peace of mind. We'll explore the delicious world of fresh, whole foods, and dig into the art of harmonizing tastes and textures, all while keeping your migraine triggers at away.

Whether you're a seasoned chef or just starting your culinary journey, these recipes are meant to be accessible and simple to follow. We've provided extensive directions, useful recommendations, and nutritional information to assist you every step of the way. Moreover, our recipes embrace a broad variety of dietary needs, including vegan, gluten-free, and low-sodium alternatives, so everyone may appreciate the delight of eating without concern.

So, if you're ready to take charge of your migraine journey and go on a tasty adventure, join us as we explore a world of wonderful, migraine-friendly foods. Say goodbye to migraine triggers and welcome to tasty, healthy recipes that feed your body and spirit. Welcome to a brighter, pain-free future with Migraine-Friendly Recipes!

GRILLED SALMON WITH LEMON AND HERBS

Ingredients:

- Salmon fillets
- Lemon juice
- Fresh herbs (such as thyme, rosemary, or dill)
- Olive oil
- Salt and pepper

Instructions:

- Preheat the grill to medium-high heat.
- Brush salmon fillets with olive oil, sprinkle with herbs, and season with salt & pepper.
- Grill for roughly 4-5 minutes each side or until the fish flakes easily. Drizzle with lemon juice before serving.

QUINOA SALAD WITH ROASTED VEGETABLES

Ingredients:

- Quinoa

- Assorted roasted veggies (bell peppers, zucchini, cherry tomatoes, etc.)
- Olive oil
- Balsamic vinegar
- Fresh basil
- Salt and pepper

Instructions:
- Cook quinoa according to package directions.
- Toss roasted veggies with olive oil, balsamic vinegar, basil, salt, and pepper.
- Serve the quinoa topped with the roasted veggies.

CHICKEN AND VEGETABLE STIR-FRY

Ingredients:
- Chicken breast or tofu
- Assorted veggies (broccoli, bell peppers, snap peas, carrots, etc.)
- Low-sodium soy sauce or tamari
- Ginger and garlic

- Sesame oil
- Brown rice or cauliflower rice (for serving)

Instructions:

- Cook chicken or tofu in a skillet with a little sesame oil until cooked through.
- Stir-fry the veggies until they're tender-crisp.
- Combine cooked protein and veggies, then add soy sauce, ginger, and garlic for flavor.
- Serve over brown rice or cauliflower rice.

SPINACH AND FETA STUFFED CHICKEN

Ingredients:

- Chicken breasts
- Fresh spinach
- Feta cheese
- Garlic powder
- Paprika
- Olive oil
- Salt and pepper

Instructions:
- Preheat oven to 375°F (190°C).
- Butterfly chicken breasts and fill with spinach and crumbled feta cheese.
- Sprinkle with garlic powder, paprika, salt, and pepper.
- Drizzle with olive oil and bake for 25-30 minutes or until chicken is cooked through.

MANGO AND AVOCADO SALAD

Ingredients:
- Ripe mango
- Avocado
- Red onion
- Fresh cilantro
- Lime juice
- Salt and pepper

Instructions:
- Dice mango and avocado.
- Finely slice red onion and cilantro.
- Toss all ingredients together and sprinkle with lime juice. Season with salt and pepper.

BAKED SWEET POTATO FRIES

Ingredients:

- Sweet potatoes
- Olive oil
- Paprika
- Cumin
- Salt

Instructions:

- Preheat oven to 425°F (220°C).
- Cut sweet potatoes into fries, and sprinkle with olive oil, paprika, cumin, and salt.
- Bake for 25-30 minutes or until crispy, turning halfway through.

LENTIL AND VEGETABLE SOUP

Ingredients:

- Green or brown lentils
- Assorted veggies (carrots, celery, onion, etc.)
- Low-sodium vegetable broth
- Bay leaves
- Thyme
- Salt and pepper

Instructions:

- Sauté veggies until softened, then add lentils, vegetable broth, bay leaves, thyme, salt, and pepper.
- Simmer until lentils are cooked, approximately 25-30 minutes.

TURKEY AND CRANBERRY LETTUCE WRAPS

Ingredients:

- Ground turkey
- Cranberries
- Lettuce leaves
- Walnuts
- Cinnamon
- Salt and pepper

Instructions:

- Cook ground turkey until browned, then add cranberries, chopped walnuts, cinnamon, salt, and pepper.
- Spoon the mixture onto lettuce leaves for a delicious wrap.

GREEK YOGURT PARFAIT

Ingredients:

- Greek yogurt
- Fresh berries (blueberries, strawberries, raspberries)
- Honey
- Granola (optional)

Instructions:

- Layer Greek yogurt, fresh berries, and a sprinkle of honey in a glass.
- Add granola for added crunch if desired.

ZUCCHINI NOODLES WITH PESTO

Ingredients:

- Zucchini noodles (zoodles)
- Homemade or store-bought pesto
- Cherry tomatoes
- Pine nuts (optional)

Instructions:

- Sauté zucchini noodles till tender.
- Toss with pesto and halved cherry tomatoes.
- Sprinkle with pine nuts if desired.

OATMEAL WITH ALMOND BUTTER AND BANANAS

Ingredients:

- Rolled oats
- Almond butter
- Bananas
- Cinnamon
- Honey (optional)

Instructions:

- Cook oats according to package directions.
- Top with almond butter, sliced bananas, a sprinkling of cinnamon, and a drizzle of honey if preferred.

ROASTED BEET AND GOAT CHEESE SALAD

Ingredients:

- Roasted beets
- Mixed greens
- Goat cheese
- Toasted walnuts
- Balsamic vinaigrette

Instructions:

- Toss mixed greens with roasted beets, crumbled goat cheese, and toasted walnuts.
- Drizzle with balsamic vinaigrette.

SALMON AND ASPARAGUS FOIL PACKETS

Ingredients:

- Salmon fillets
- Asparagus spears
- Lemon slices
- Dill
- Olive oil
- Salt and pepper

Instructions:

- Place fish and asparagus on a piece of foil.
- Top with lemon slices, dill, olive oil, salt, and pepper.
- Seal the foil package and bake at 400°F (200°C) for approximately 15-20 minutes.

TURKEY AND VEGETABLE STUFFED BELL PEPPERS

Ingredients:
- Bell peppers
- Ground turkey
- Quinoa
- Diced tomatoes
- Onion
- Garlic
- Italian seasoning
- Salt and pepper

Instructions:
- Cut the tops off bell peppers and remove the seeds.
- Cook ground turkey, quinoa, chopped tomatoes, onion, garlic, Italian seasoning, salt, and pepper.
- Stuff the peppers with the mixture and bake at 375°F (190°C) for approximately 30-35 minutes.

CUCUMBER AND MINT GAZPACHO

Ingredients:
- Cucumbers

- Greek yogurt
- Fresh mint
- Garlic
- Lemon juice
- Salt and pepper

Instructions:

- Blend cucumbers, Greek yogurt, fresh mint, garlic, lemon juice, salt, and pepper until smooth.
- Chill and serve as a delightful cold soup.

BAKED CHICKEN TENDERS WITH ALMOND FLOUR

Ingredients:

- Chicken tenders
- Almond flour
- Paprika
- Garlic powder
- Egg (for dipping)

Instructions:

- Dip chicken tenders in beaten egg, then cover with a combination of

almond flour, paprika, and garlic powder.
- Bake at 400°F (200°C) until crispy and cooked through.

MASHED CAULIFLOWER

Ingredients:
- Cauliflower florets
- Butter or olive oil
- Garlic powder
- Salt and pepper

Instructions:
- Steam cauliflower until soft, then mash with butter or olive oil, garlic powder, salt, and pepper.

BALSAMIC GLAZED CHICKEN

Ingredients:
- Chicken breasts
- Balsamic vinegar
- Brown sugar or honey
- Garlic
- Rosemary
- Salt and pepper

Instructions:

- Sear chicken breasts, then simmer in a combination of balsamic vinegar, brown sugar or honey, garlic, rosemary, salt, and pepper until cooked through.

STIR-FRIED TOFU WITH BROCCOLI AND CASHEWS

Ingredients:

- Tofu
- Broccoli florets
- Cashews
- Low-sodium soy sauce or tamari
- Ginger and garlic
- Sesame oil
- Brown rice or cauliflower rice (for serving)

Instructions:

- Press tofu to remove extra moisture, then stir-fry with broccoli, cashews, soy sauce, ginger, garlic, and sesame oil.

- Serve over brown rice or cauliflower rice.

OVEN-ROASTED BRUSSEL SPROUTS

Ingredients:

- Brussel sprouts
- Olive oil
- Balsamic vinegar
- Garlic powder
- Salt and pepper

Instructions:

- Toss Brussels sprouts with olive oil, balsamic vinegar, garlic powder, salt, and pepper.
- Roast in the oven at 400°F (200°C) until crispy and caramelized.

WEIGHT MANAGEMENT: UNLOCKING THE KEY TO MIGRAINE RELIEF

In a culture that frequently appears preoccupied with looks and numbers on a scale, the notion of weight control is surely a subject of universal interest. Beyond aesthetics, weight management has a deep impact on our entire health and well-being, with links that transcend into unforeseen realms. One such area of curiosity is the complicated relationship between weight, obesity, and migraines.

Migraines, those terrible headaches typically accompanied by nausea, light sensitivity, and throbbing pain, have long been the topic of scientific research. A recent study has exposed a remarkable association between migraine frequency and weight. While migraines themselves are diverse, comprising a complex interaction of genetics, environment, and neurological variables, it turns out that your body weight may have a more substantial influence on migraine incidence than you may assume.

So, let's start on a thrilling trip to examine the relationship between weight, obesity, and migraines, and learn how weight management measures might serve as a beacon of hope for people seeking relief from these terrible headaches.

The Weighty Connection: Obesity and Migraines
Imagine a seesaw where, on one side, there's extra physical weight, and on the other, there's a load of migraines. The balance between these two parameters may be delicate, and tilting it in favor of weight control may hold the secret to migraine relief.

Obesity, defined as an excessive buildup of body fat, is a well-known risk factor for various health disorders, including heart disease, diabetes, and sleep apnea. However, it's the relationship between fat and migraines that has been getting growing attention.

Studies have revealed that persons with obesity are more prone to develop chronic migraines, defined as headaches occurring on 15 or more days per month. The reasons underlying this relationship are various. Adipose tissue, usually referred to as fat, isn't simply a passive storage unit; it's metabolically active and generates numerous hormones and inflammatory compounds. These bioactive substances may impact brain chemistry and provoke migraine episodes.

Furthermore, obesity is related to other comorbid problems such as sleep apnea and insulin resistance, which may increase migraine frequency and intensity. It's like a domino effect, when one health condition topples into another, producing a vicious cycle that might feel insurmountable.

Weight Management: A Light at the End of the Tunnel
Now that we've studied the labyrinthine relationship between weight and migraines, the question arises: how might weight

management measures come to the rescue? The good news is that taking control of your weight isn't only about dropping pounds for looks; it's about restoring your health and maybe easing migraine misery.

Lifestyle Modifications: The cornerstone of weight control is adopting a healthy lifestyle. This involves regular physical exercise, a balanced diet, and stress management. Engaging in cardiovascular sports like walking, swimming, or cycling will not only help you lose extra weight but also lower the frequency and severity of migraine episodes.

Nutritional Awareness: Paying attention to your food is crucial. Identifying and eliminating trigger foods such as aged cheese, processed meats, and artificial sweeteners may help control migraines. Additionally, maintaining stable blood sugar levels by eating frequent meals and keeping hydrated helps avoid headaches.

Medication and Support: Sometimes, weight control involves medical intervention. Healthcare practitioners might prescribe drugs to promote weight reduction, particularly when other health issues like diabetes or hypertension are present. Seeking help from healthcare experts, dietitians, and support groups may be important on your weight control journey.

Sleep Hygiene: Adequate and restful sleep is vital for both weight control and migraine prevention. Establishing a regular sleep regimen and managing sleep problems like sleep apnea may make a substantial impact.

Mind-Body Practices: Practices like mindfulness meditation and yoga may help control stress, a recognized cause of migraines. These strategies may help build a healthy connection with food and eating, leading to successful weight control.

Conclusion: A Brighter Future Awaits

Weight management isn't only a cosmetic task; it's a lifeline for individuals suffering the merciless grip of migraines. By tackling weight and adopting healthy lifestyle choices, you may tilt the seesaw in favor of well-being and find relief from these terrible headaches. Remember, the route to weight control is a marathon, not a sprint, but the rewards—a healthy body and fewer migraines—are surely worth the effort. So, embrace this trip, and a happier, migraine-free future awaits on the other side.